TRANSACTIONS

OF THE

AMERICAN PHILOSOPHICAL SOCIETY

HELD AT PHILADELPHIA

FOR PROMOTING USEFUL KNOWLEDGE

NEW SERIES—VOLUME 62, PART 1
1972

MAURUS OF SALERNO

Twelfth-century "Optimus Physicus"

With his Commentary on the Prognostics of Hippocrates

*Now first transcribed from manuscript and
translated into English by*

MORRIS HAROLD SAFFRON, M.D.

Lecturer in Medical History, Rutgers Medical School

THE AMERICAN PHILOSOPHICAL SOCIETY
INDEPENDENCE SQUARE
PHILADELPHIA

January, 1972

Library of Congress Catalog
Card Number 78-184164

ISBN 0-87169-621-5

FOREWORD

An early interest in the history of medieval medicine, reawakened by the reading of Loren MacKinney's scholarly lectures, was intensified when I finally managed to acquire a pristine set of the *Collectio Salernitana*, one which had obviously never been opened, much less read. Then began a timid incursion into the formidable pages of this poorly printed work and a gradually increasing familiarity with the medical language of the texts. To improve my background in medieval studies I returned to Columbia University for courses in the history, philosophy, and literature of the period, all of which led eventually to a seminar under Professor Lynn Thorndike of revered memory.

It was at this point, some twenty years ago, that Professor Paul Oskar Kristeller first suggested that I transcribe and edit the present text, but the work proved difficult and tedious, and was all too frequently interrupted by the demands of an active medical practice. I need not emphasize my indebtedness to Professor Kristeller, not only for his personal encouragement and advice, but for the benefit all medical historians have derived from his illuminating papers on the School of Salerno.

To Professor William D. Sharpe of the New Jersey College of Medicine, I owe a special debt of gratitude, one which it is a great pleasure to acknowledge. He has helped me in many ways: by checking the final drafts of my texts, both Latin and English, by suggesting definite pathologic entities for the obscure disease processes mentioned by Maurus, by meticulous care in proofreading the typescript, and—what is perhaps most important—by relentlessly urging me on to complete the work.

I am also grateful to Professor Pearl Kibre of Hunter College, University of the City of New York, for many kindnesses. In the 1963 revision of Thorndike and Kibre she noted that the present work was in progress. From the incipits of B. N. lat. 18499 which I had supplied, Dr. Kibre was able to identify two related manuscripts: one, Vatican lat. 4477, containing an expanded, probably later, version of Maurus' Commentary on the Prognostics; the other, B. N. lat. 7102, containing only the prologue. I found the Vatican text useful in clarifying certain textual ambiguities and in confirming certain conjectures as to the correct meaning of several textual corruptions in B. N. lat. 18499.

Then I would be indeed remiss were I not to express my sincere thanks to several librarian friends, and especially to Miss Gertrude Annan, Mrs. Alice D. Weaver, and Mrs. Sali W. Morganstern of the New York Academy of Medicine who never wearied in supplying my countless requests. I thank also Frederick B. Goff of the Library of Congress, John B. Blake of the National Library of Medicine, Kenneth B. Lohf of the Columbia University Libraries, and the authorities of the Bibliothèque Nationale and the Vatican Library for much needed information.

Of the many Salernitan works already in print, only a handful have achieved translation into modern languages. In English, I know only of the versions of the anatomical treatises prepared by Dr. George W. Corner, who very kindly sent me reprints of several of his articles on Salerno. I hope that the present translation will in some way fill an apparent need by providing students an opportunity to come to grips directly with the thought and teachings of one of the most influential and admired masters of *Hochsalerno*.

M. H. S.

New York City

MAURUS OF SALERNO

Twelfth-century "Optimus Physicus"

With his Commentary on the Prognostics of Hippocrates

Now first transcribed from manuscript and translated into English by

MORRIS HAROLD SAFFRON, M.D.

CONTENTS

INTRODUCTION

THE SCHOOL OF SALERNO

In the revival of western medicine and science, the school of Salerno occupies a position of fundamental importance. It is true that as early as the reign of Charlemange, and continuing throughout the post-Carolingian period, serious attempts had been made to re-introduce the systematic study of medicine. The monasteries of St. Gall, Monte Cassino, Bobbio, Fulda, Lorsch, Reichenau, Fleury, and Tours, and later the cathedral schools of Rheims, Chartres, and Canterbury were but a few of the more notable centers at which a handful of texts—the *membra disiecta* of ancient medicine—were cherished, read, copied, and expounded. The importance of these early schools in preserving the medical knowledge of antiquity is quite obvious, and has been acknowledged by all historians.[1]

Nevertheless at these ecclesiastical teaching centers, devoted primarily, as they were, to the liberal arts, the course of instruction in medicine never attained a status of major importance. The medical curriculum lacked continuity and organization, and the relative prominence of a school might end abruptly with the death of a famous master. Chartres was by far the most advanced and most enduring of the cathedral schools at which medicine was seriously taught, and at its peak during the eleventh century succeeded in attracting students from as far away as England and Germany. Yet even at Chartres there is no trace of organized instruction in the practice of medicine, and indeed the great Fulbert (960–1028) makes a clear distinction between the lowly practitioner and the learned amateur who approaches medical theory as one of the liberal arts, or as an avocation, or simply as an adjunct to *physica*.[2] Because clerics were forbidden to perform surgical procedures and could obviously take no part in the practice of gynecology and obstetrics, these important subjects were relegated to the unlettered *sanguinatores* and midwives.[3] Furthermore, during the twelfth century a succession of Church councils passed increasingly stringent regulations enjoining clerics from all forms of extra-mural medical practice and

[1] Carolingian efforts at medical education are outlined by V. L. Bullough, 1966: pp. 36–37; for a detailed account of the post-Carolingian period, especially in France, see the monograph by L. C. MacKinney, 1937. Still useful are two older works by G. F. Fort, 1883: chap. 11 and 14; and T. Puschmann, 1891: pp. 183–196. For the content of the surviving literature see H. E. Sigerist, "The Latin Medical Literature," *Jour. Hist. Med.* **13** (1958): pp. 127–146. as well as the fundamental study by A. Beccaria, 1956.

[2] D. Reisman, 1936: p. 35 notes the poor opinion held by John of Salisbury (d. 1180) of the quality of education and ethical standards at the medical schools of Salerno and Montpellier. These remarks of the bishop of Chartres confirm the intense rivalry which existed between these centers.

[3] B. Lawn, 1963: p. 53 notes that William of Conches who taught at Chartres about 1125 refused to lecture on sexual matters, lest they "offend the ears of monks." This attitude contrasts strongly with that of Gilles de Corbeil, who, less than a century later, had no qualms about publishing his devastating *Hierapigra ad Prelatos*.

teaching. The growing attraction of city universities hastened the decline of the cathedral schools, and the beginning of systematic medical instruction at Paris during the closing decades of the twelfth century led to the final exodus of medical students and their masters from Chartres.[4]

If the relative freedom and intellectual ferment of city life were in fact essential to a revival of interest in medical studies, then the bustling town of Salerno on the Gulf of Paestum, astride the pilgrim and crusader routes between east and west, undoubtedly provided elements particularly favorable for such a development. The healthy climate and mineral springs, already famous in antiquity, continued to draw chronic invalids to this seaside resort, while a close association with the schools and libraries of Monte Cassino and Benevento, the continuing contacts of Campania with Byzantium, the proximity to Sicily, an outpost of Arabic civilization, and the lingering vestiges of the language and culture of Magna Graecia, all combined to attract first an unusual concentration of physicians and, by the eleventh century, a growing number of medical students.[5] Certainly the physicians of Salerno led the West in the cultivation of medicine as a separate discipline. The dim and uncertain origins of this celebrated school have for centuries intrigued romantic antiquarians as well as serious historians, and a host of uncritical writers have helped to perpetuate the school's legendary history.[6]

The first scholarly account of the medical school of Salerno appeared in 1790, but the erudite Ackermann was hampered by a lack of familiarity with the Salernitan literature, most of which was still gathering dust in the libraries of Europe. It was not until Henschel, Daremberg, and other scholars made their remarkable series of discoveries in the mid-nineteenth century that the truly formidable size of the Salernitan medical corpus gradually became apparent. The task of transcribing and printing the newly discovered texts was accomplished primarily through the efforts of Salvatore DeRenzi, whose *Collectio Salernitana*,[7]

although occasionally marred by inadequacies, remains the indispensable source. Later writers, including Giacosa,[8] Garufi,[9] and Capparoni[10] added historical or textual data of the greatest significance.

The next impetus to Salernitan studies came from Karl Sudhoff and his school. Sudhoff evinced an unusual affinity not only for Salerno but for Maurus himself, calling him "the leading spokesman of the school of Salerno as anatomist, teacher and pathfinding clinician."[11] He encouraged three of his students to edit works of Maurus, namely the *Anatomia Mauri*,[12] the *De Flebotomia*,[13] and the *De Urinis*.[14] Among Sudhoff's followers, Creutz and Sigerist in particular continued to make valuable contributions to the study of Salerno, and for a Sudhoff *Festschrift*, the Singers wrote an illuminating article on the origins and early literature of the school.[15] Two American scholars have also contributed significantly. Corner wrote the still standard account of the development of anatomy at Salerno and several papers on Salernitan medicine and surgery, and he may well have been the first scholar in recent times to mention our manuscript (B. N. lat. 18499).[16] Kristeller, who was attracted to Salerno as an early recipient of the "new" Aristotle, wrote a fundamental paper in 1945 and followed this with several others. He refuted unwarranted claims as to the antiquity of the *collegium*, criticized loose use of the expression "School of Salerno," studied the introduction of the term *physicus*, traced the development of the *Articella* and described the earliest known Salernitan commentaries on that collection.[17]

---

[4] Monastic and cathedral school medicine is well documented in L. Dubreuil-Chambardel, 1914, especially chap. 15. For Chartres see J. Tribalet, 1936, as well as MacKinney, chap. 3 and Bullough, pp. 40–45, 49–52 and 114–115 (bibliography). The conciliar decisions affecting the clerical practice of medicine are usefully tabulated by Riesman, pp. 23–24.

[5] W. Artelt, "Die Salernoforschung," *Sudhoffs Archiv* 40 (1956): pp. 211–230 gives a full account of studies in Salernitan historiography during the past three centuries.

[6] J. C. G. Ackermann, *Regimen Sanitatis Salerni* (Stendal, 1790), preserves the early, traditional accounts of the school's origin.

[7] S. DeRenzi, *Collectio Salernitana* (Naples, 1852–1859, 5 v.); hereafter referred to as *CS*. As a detailed history of the school, DeRenzi's *Storia Documentata* (2nd ed., Naples, 1857) has never been superseded. A. W. E. T. Henschel (*CS* 2: pp. 1–71) gives a full account of his discovery of the Breslau codex (1837), the cornerstone of Salernitan studies. Creutz and Steudel, 1949: p. 130 conclude that the codex was compiled by two Salernitans between 1160 and 1170.

[8] P. Giacosa, *Magistri Salernitani nondum editi* (Turin, 1901, 2 v.), a remarkable collection of texts and documents unknown to DeRenzi. The second volume contains photographic plates of manuscripts.

[9] C. A. Garufi, *Necrologio del Liber Confratrum di S. Matteo di Salerno* (Rome, 1922), an important source of biographical data relating to the noble and professional classes of Salerno.

[10] Garufi's data pertaining particularly to physicians are conveniently excerpted by P. Capparoni, *Magistri Salernitani nondum cogniti* (London, 1923).

[11] *Archiv für die Geschichte der Medizin* 21 (1929): pp. 53, 55; *Archeion* 14: (1932) p. 363.

[12] W. L. H. Ploss, *Anatomia Mauri* (Leipzig, 1919). Other versions of this work also attributed to Maurus were edited by Corner (1927) and Sudhoff (1928).

[13] R. Buerschaper, *Ein bisher unbekannter Aderlasstraktat* (Leipzig, 1919), and see our note 92.

[14] A. Kadner (1919) translated this work into German; G. W. Corner, "The Rise of Medicine at Salerno," *Annals. Med Hist.*, n.s. 3 (1931): pp. 6–7 gives an excerpt in English translation.

[15] An excellent introductory account of Salerno is found in Creutz and Steudel, 1949: pp. 117–159. Creutz was particularly attracted to Urso, Maurus's colleague, and wrote several articles stressing Urso's importance as a philosopher-physician. Still rewarding is the paper by Charles and Dorothea Singer, "The Origin of the Medical School of Salerno, the first University," in *Essays on the History of Medicine presented to Karl Sudhoff* (Zurich, 1924), pp. 121–138.

[16] G. W. Corner, *Anatomical Texts of the Earlier Middle Ages* (Washington, 1927), especially p. 26, and see our bibliography.

[17] P. G. Kristeller, "The School of Salerno," *Bull. Hist. Med.*

During the last two decades a German scholar, Heinrich Schipperges, contributed several important papers which reconsider the entire subject of the introduction of Arabic science and medicine into Europe.[18] The Constantinian problem was included in this thorough review,[19] and new lists of Constantinius's translations and original works were prepared to supplement the century-old essay by Steinschneider.[20] At Rome, Pazzini and his school have begun the translation into Italian of selected major Salernitan works, regrettably using the often defective texts of DeRenzi instead of transcribing superior versions still in manuscript.[21] In Salerno itself, a recent revival of interest in historical studies has led to the formation of an active society and the publication of a journal.[22]

Recently, two Englishmen have approached Salerno tangentially. Lawn's masterful study, although relating primarily to the historical development of lists of questions used as teaching aids, throws considerable light on the medical and philosophical theories current in twelfth-century Salerno.[23] Talbot, in his brief but stimulating chapter on Salerno, concludes that, despite the influx of the Arabic literature, the quality of medical practice did not improve radically during the first half of the twelfth century, and that the influence of Salerno on northern European and especially on English medicine before the twelfth century has been exaggerated.[24]

Following Sudhoff it has been customary to divide the history of Salerno into three convenient periods, but Creutz's modification of Sudhoff's original scheme seems preferable:

900–1100　Early, Pre-Constantinian
1100–1225　*Hochsalerno*, The "Great" Period
1225–1400　Late, Post-Neapolitan, The Period of
　　　　　　　Decline

Little is definitely known of early Salerno.[25] The rising fame of the town as a medical center is implied in Richer's tale of a ninth-century Salernitan physician at the French court, and by the visits of such celebrated patients as Adalbero, bishop of Verdun, and Desiderius, abbot of Monte Cassino.[26] DeRenzi collected the names of sixteen physicians who practiced at Salerno before 1050,[27] and among these, at least two deserve our attention: Gariopontus (*ca.* 1035) is noted for his *Passionarius Galeni*, a handbook of pathology and therapeutics compiled from the residual writings of late classical and Byzantine medicine;[28] and the quasilegendary Petrocellus, whose *Practica* is a work of the same derivative character.[29] At almost the same period flourished the physician-bishop Alfanus (*ob.* 1085), who demonstrated the vitality of the Greek tradition by translating the περὶ φύσεος ἀνθρώπου of Nemesius.[30] One additional

17 (1945): pp. 138–194; reissued with additions in *Studies in Renaissance Thoughts and Letters* (Rome, 1956): pp. 495–551, and in Italian translation in *Rassegna Storica Salernitana*, Anno XVI–XVII (Salerno, 1955–1956). For additional studies on Salerno by Kristeller see our bibliography.

18 For Schipperges's encyclopedic and stimulating studies, see our bibliography. An English translation would be most desirable.

19 Schipperges, 1955: pp. 62–68; 1964: pp. 17–49.

20 M. Steinschneider, "Constantinus Africanus und seine Arabische Quellen," *Virchows Archiv* 31, (1866): pp 351–410. This fundamental study has never been superseded.

21 Compare the *copia imperfetta* of Maurus' *Commentary on the Aphorisms* (*Storia Documentata*, p. 333) with the superior version in our MS (B.N. lat. 18499: ff. 55vA–122vB).

22 The Centro di Studi di Medicina Medioevale, founded in 1952, is associated with the L'Archivo di Stato di Salerno. A periodical *Salerno Hippocratica Civitas*, which first appeared in 1967 is devoted to the medical history of the community and is sponsored by the Comitate Permanente per la Risorgente Scuola Medica Salernitana.

23 Brian Lawn, *The Salernitan Questions* (Oxford, 1963). I am greatly indebted to this brillant study, although I cannot follow Lawn's chronology of the career of Gilles de Corbeil.

24 G. H. Talbot, 1967: pp. 18, 45–47, follows the thesis of K. Bloedner, 1925, in considering the Petrocellus text to be derived from a non-Salernitan prototype which circulated widely throughout Italy and northern Europe. Nevertheless, the affinities between the *Peri Didaxeon* and the Petrocellus *Practica* seem too close to be explained by a common ancestor. See also J. F. Payne, 1904: pp. 142–167, and Grattan and Singer, 1952: pp. 75–79. Kristeller (personal communication) believes that considerable Salernitan influence on early English medicine can be inferred by the many Salernitan MSS which have survived in English libraries since medieval times.

25 The heated discussions between Puccinotti and DeRenzi as to monastic *versus* lay influences on the origin of Salerno seem to have ended in compromise. There was undoubtedly some Benedictine encouragement, but the school was predominantly lay from the beginning. For DeRenzi's final rebuttal of the monastic thesis, see Francesco Puccinotti, *Storia della Medicina* (Naples, 1860–1863, 2 v.) 1: pp. 373–388. Among contemporary historians Pazzini still veers to the monastic origin, although holding a "giudizio ragionevolmente eclettico fra i due precedenti autori," 1962: p. 180.

26 Fort, pp. 229–230, 233–234, reports the Richer tale in considerable detail, and mentions the famous visitors to Salerno.

27 *Storia Documentata*, pp. 156, 188; although DeRenzi lists several Hebrew-speaking physicians he fails to mention Donnolo, for whom see Steinschneider (1867) and H. Friedenwald, *The Jews and Medicine* (Baltimore, 1944–1946, 2 v.) 1: pp. 148–152.

28 Among the sources clearly identified are the Aurelius-Aesculapius text, the Galenic *Epistula ad Glauconem* and Theodore Priscian (Beccaria, pp. 35–36). The first two works formed part of an eighth-century *Summa*, the existence of which was originally postulated by Giacosa, p. xxvi, and recently defined more precisely by Lawn, pp. 6–7. In the *Passionarius* of Gariopontus, long attributed to Galen himself, are also to be noted selections from Paul of Aegina and Alexander of Tralles (Giacosa, p. xxvii), as well as extracts from *noster Hippocrates*. In our own text Maurus refers to the *Passionarius* only once (15.9), yet the remarkable popularity of this work is attested by three early sixteenth century editions. (R. J. Durling, 1967: p. 242).

29 Kadner, p. 46; Pazzini, in the Introduction to *Mauro Salernitano, Commentario agli Aforismi di Ippocrate*, Luigi Stroppiana and Renato Minghetti, trans. (Rome, 1959), pp. 19–21 expresses a generally poor opinion of this work, going so far as to question the attribution to Maurus. He regards certain parallels with the Petrocellus text as suggestive of their common ignorance of historical fact. See also our note 3 to the text of the Commentary.

30 For Nemesius (*fl.* A.D. late fourth century) see E. Skard,

late-eleventh-century compilation is also known, the famous *Antidotarium Nicolai*, the earliest prototype of the European pharmacopoeia.[31]

These eleventh-century compilations are marked by a severely practical, didactic tone, and were undoubtedly intended as authoritative texts in the instruction of an ever-increasing number of students. They remained basic requirements of the curriculum throughout the first half of the twelfth century, and were only gradually supplemented or replaced by the texts of the *Articella*.[32]

It was long thought that the early medieval physician had access to a very restricted library, and that the writings translated from the Arabic by Constantinus Africanus from 1077 to 1087 came as a complete revelation to the physicians of Salerno. Our views on this subject have been greatly modified by the work of Giacosa (1901) and Singer (1917). Kibre (1945) showed the wide dispersion of the Hippocratic writings during the early Middle Ages,[33] and Beccaria (1956) published his indispensable census, listing no fewer than 117 surviving medical manuscripts which antedate 1100. Of these, at least fifteen, of the very highest quality, are in the local Beneventan script.[34] Among the writings thus circulating were such classics as the *Aphorisms* and *Prognostics* of Hippocrates, the former with Galen's commentary, Galen's *Ars parva* with the *Isagoge* of Johannitius; as well as works of Alexander of Tralles, Priscian, Oribasius, Paul of Aegina, Antonius Musa, Apuleius, Caelius Aurelianus, Cassius Felix, and

Isidore of Seville. Salerno shows no direct knowledge of Celsus, although three early medieval manuscripts of the *De medicina* are now known to exist. One author insists that much of the material common to Celsus and other early writers may have come to Salerno through Paul of Aegina.[35]

Because of our more accurate insight into the quantity and quality of the medical literature already available at Salerno before Constantinius's arrival (*ca.* 1075), we are now in a better position to understand why the translations from the Arabic failed to produce—at least immediately—so profound an effect as was formerly thought. By 1100, when the first of these foreign works made their appearance at Salerno, the school was rapidly attaining recognition as the foremost medical center in Europe, students were pouring in from the northernmost reaches of the continent, and an atmosphere of satisfied parochialism must have pervaded the association of masters in the self-styled *Civitas Hippocratica*. There can be little doubt that at least as far as therapy was concerned, the cautious and practical Salernitans deliberately resisted the disturbing innovations from abroad, loath to admit that their *Passionarius* and *Antidotarium* could be improved upon. Scalinci, for example, flatly denies any influence of Constantinus on the oculists of Salerno.[36]

Nevertheless, among the thirty-seven translations attributed to Constantinus by Steinschneider were many distinguished works, including the *Pantegni* of Haly-Abbas, the *Viaticum* of Ibn-Jazzar and the treatises on diets, fevers, and urine of Isaac Judaeus, and these undoubtedly enabled the Salernitans to extend their intellectual horizon. Anatomy and pathology, hitherto little studied at Salerno, received increasing attention: thus, the primitive anatomical demonstration attributed to Copho (*ca.* 1100) shows only traces of Arabic influence, whereas the second, quite possibly by Bartholomaeus (*ca.* 1120), borrows almost literally from the *Pantegni* and—what is perhaps even more important—indicates demonstrable familiarity with early scholastic apparatus and methodology.[37]

1940: pp. 562–566. The eleventh century Salernitan writers are discussed briefly by G. Sarton, *Introduction*: 1927: 1: pp. 725–727. The remarkable Alfanus, poet, book-collector, archbishop and physician, provides a direct link between Monte Cassino and Salerno. His translation of the *Premnon Physicon* of Nemesius brought to the West much material stemming directly from Galen, and had a wide influence on Salerno and northern Europe (Lawn, pp. 18, 22). In the scant half-century separating Alfanus and Maurus Greek learning at Salerno must have declined rapidly.

[31] The traditional attribution of this immensely popular work to an unidentified Niccolò has recently been questioned by Ongaro, 1968: pp. 40–42. He argues rather convincingly that the text of the printed editions may well be a product of the thirteenth century. There are no fewer than thirteen incunables (Klebs, 1963: p. 243) as well as several sixteenth-century editions (Durling, p. 429). A modern critical edition is that of Paul Dorveaux (1906).

[32] The thirteenth-century Bartholomaeus-Musandinus manuscript of the *Articella*, first described in full by Kristeller (*Nuove Fonti*, pp. 63–64), but as yet unpublished, is still accompanied by the glosses of Platearius on the *Antidotarium*; Friedenwald 1: p. 192 owned another thirteenth-century *Articella* manuscript (now in Jerusalem) which includes four treatises by Isaac Judaeus. Apparently these works were soon dropped from the canon because they do not appear in any of the printed editions of the *Articella*.

[33] P. Kibre, "Hippocratic Writings in the Middle Ages," *Bull. Hist. Med.* 18 (1945): pp. 371–412. Since this important article appeared Dr. Kibre has accumulated much additional material, now being prepared for publication.

[34] Beccaria, 1956: p. 58 discusses the manuscript in Beneventan script.

[35] See N. Scalinci, 1941: pp. 134–135, where he quotes as one authority DeRenzi. The latter, while preparing his own edition of Celsus (Naples, 1851), satisfied himself that there were numerous parallels between Celsus and Paul of Aegina. D. De Moulin, 1964: p. 30 also asserts that Celsus was better known in the early Middle Ages than is usually supposed.

[36] Scalinci, p. 149; Adelard of Bath, the English student of *physica* who spent some time at Salerno after the Constantinian translations had become freely available there seems to have made little use of these in preparing his own list of scientific questions. On the other hand, the influence of Nemesius through Alfanus is still readily discernible in the *Quaestiones Naturales* (Lawn, pp. 24–25).

[37] Corner (*Anatomical Texts*, p. 25) shows that the anonymous author of this second anatomical demonstration had already written commentaries on Johannitius, Philaretus and the *Aphorisms* of Hippocrates. Through his examination of our manuscript (B. N. lat. 18499), Corner eliminated Maurus as a

It may well have been this same Bartholomaeus who first selected from the mass of Constantinian translations those works he considered best adapted for assimilation at Salerno.[38] The texts included in the earliest versions of the *Articella* were carefully chosen to blend with the so-called Galenic tradition of the school, and thus enabled such later conservatives as Matthew Platearius and Musandinus[39] to offer some resistance to Arabic infiltration. That the full impact of these Arabic works was not entirely beneficial has been shown by Talbot, who finds that the *De aegritudinum curatione*[40]—a composite work written by seven masters (including Bartholomaeus) sometime before 1150—demonstrates little advance on the century-old Gariopontus and Petrocellus texts, and in its reliance on Arabic charms, polypharmacy, and *Dreckapotheke* actually indicates a regression.[41]

There is nevertheless universal agreement that the twelfth century witnessed the peak of Salernitan achievement, and indeed Haskins relied heavily on Salerno in support of his well-known thesis.[42] Under a succession of enlightened Norman kings, city life became secure and prosperous, and a series of drastic laws regulating the practice of medicine (1140) made quackery an unprofitable occupation. Regardless of the other effects Constantinus may have had on Salerno, the threat of his translations undoubtedly served to stimulate the Salernitan masters to increased literary activity, perhaps in self-defense.[43] Certainly from 1100 onward, the profusion of indigenous writings becomes quite remarkable. As already indicated, the first half of the century is dominated by the figure of Bartholomaeus who, like his predecessors Copho and John Platearius, was author of a famous *Practica*. A man of intellectual vigor, Bartholomaeus is of particular interest to us as quite possibly the first physician in the medieval west to undertake an original series of commentaries on such revered masters as Hippocrates and Galen.[44]

For the student of twelfth-century Salerno, the writings of Gilles de Corbeil are a source of unusual importance.[45] In particular, they contain several revealing references to Maurus which are fundamental to any reconstruction of the master's life. Gilles, who seems to have been born about 1140, came to Paris as a youth to study logic with Adam du Petit Pont, and sometime after Adam's death (*ca.* 1159), departed for Salerno. At the time of his arrival, Bartholomaeus was no longer alive, Matthew Platearius, though living, was no longer active, but the aging Musandinus (*ob. ca.* 1165) still remained at the peak of his powers. Although Gilles regarded Musandinus as unquestionably the greatest of all his teachers, he also frequently expressed his admiration for a group of younger masters which included Maurus, Salernus, Romualdus, and Urso. Gilles continued his studies during the transition period which saw Maurus become titular head of the school,

possible author, thus leaving Bartholomaeus as a likely candidate, especially in light of the Bartholomaeus-Musandinus commentaries on these very texts now known to exist (see our note 31 above). Among the works attributed to Bartholomaeus (or Bartholomaeus Salernitanus) in Thorndike and Kibre, Col. 1758, are an *Anatomia*, commentaries on the *Aphorisms* of Hippocrates and the *Tegni* of Galen, and *Dicta* on the *Prognostics* of Hippocrates, a *Practica*, and an *Epistula ad Regem Francorom*.

[38] However, there is still no conclusive evidence that the grouping of texts to form the *Articella* actually originated at Salerno. Kristeller has found two twelfth-century commentaries on the *Articella* which seem to have no connection with Salerno, and may well derive from Chartres (*Nuove Fonti*, p. 68).

[39] Matthew Platearius was author of the *Liber de simplici medicini*, commonly known as *Circa instans*, the most influential book on materia medica and therapeutics of the Middle Ages (see Paul Dorveaux, *Le Livre des Simples Medecines* [Paris 1913]). Matthew also revised the *Antidotarium Nicolai*, adding a set of glosses which soon became more famous than the original work, and must be regarded as one of the earliest of the Salernitan commentaries. Until the discovery of the Bartholomaeus-Musandinus commentaries, the latter master was known chiefly by a small but highly regarded tract, *De cibis et potibus* (*CS* 5: pp. 254–268), which shows no suggestion of Arabic influence. It is now known that the name of Musandinus can be associated with at least eight additional works (Thorndike and Kibre, col. 1883). Of especial interest to us are the five manuscripts of Musandinus's commentary on the *Prognostics*, listed in cols. 1277 and 1619. Until these have been studied, it is obvious that the question of Maurus's originality in our own test cannot be settled.

[40] *CS* 2: pp. 81–386.

[41] Talbot, pp. 41–42.

[42] See the many references to Salerno in C. H. Haskins, *The Renaissance of the Twelfth Century* (Cambridge, Massachusetts, 1927), especially pp. 322–324.

[43] Most of the extant Salernitan literature still in manuscript or in the printed repositories was produced in the twelfth century. The question as to just how great an impact the Constantinian translations exerted on Salerno before 1150 has not yet been satisfactorily resolved. Schipperges, the most recent student of the subject, takes a negative position, considering only that Constantinus's influence was "of some weight" (1959: p. 70). He prefers the term *assimilation* to *reception* to describe the manner whereby Salerno reacted to the new learning (1964: pp. 53–54). Schipperges no longer accepts Sudhoff's description of Constantinus as "master of the Orient," but sees him much as did Charles Daremberg a century earlier as "a voice almost without an echo," (1870: 1: p. 261). Schipperges also asserts that Constantinus had "no strategic influence" on the schools of northern Europe, again reasserting the opinion expressed years before by Dubreuil-Chambardel and Wickersheimer, 1921: pp. 70–75.

[44] Talbot, p. 40, agrees that although Constantinus is often quoted, early twelfth-century Salerno still leaned heavily on Gariopontus, especially in therapeutics. At the same time, he has scant praise for the *Practice* of Bartholomaeus (*CS* 4: pp. 321–406) pointing to a profound lack of originality. Yet there are more than a dozen manuscripts of this influential work still extant (Thorndike-Kibre, cols. 773, 1080, 1785).

[45] For a brief sketch of Gilles's life, see Ernest Wickersheimer, (Paris, 1936) 1: pp. 196–197; for more extended accounts, see, C. Vieillard, *L'Urologie et les Médecins urologues dans la Médecine ancienna* (Paris, 1903), pp. 210–265 and the same author's *Gilles de Corbeil: Médecin de Philippe-Auguste et Chanoine de Notre-Dame* (Paris, 1908). I frequently refer to this excellent biography rather than to Choulant's edition of Gilles's verses as being perhaps more accessible.

and finally left Salerno after spending almost two decades there.[46]

On his homeward journey he stopped off briefly at the rival school of Montpellier, presumably to teach, but his brash advocacy of Musandinus's old-fashioned Galenic doctrines at a center already deeply committed to Arabic medicine[47] brought him a beating and expulsion. Returning to Paris about 1175, he soon opened a school in his own home, perhaps near Adam's old quarters at the Petit Pont,[48] and it was there that he wrote for the benefit of his students the *De pulsibus* and *De urinis*, metrical versions of two basic Salternitan texts. It was at this very time that Alexander Neckham, then studying with Adam of Balsham at the Petit Pont, could have heard Gilles lecture on "Hippocrates cum Galieno," that is, on texts of Hippocrates with the commentaries of Galen which Gilles had brought back with him from Italy. The close association of these two men would account for the unusual familiarity shown by Neckham with the teachings of Salerno and the contents of the *Articella*.[49]

On the other hand, Neckham's close friend and fellow-Englishman, Alfred of Sareshel, not only speaks disdainfully of the *physici* of Salerno, but in his work *De motu cordis*, makes Aristotle rather than Hippocrates the great authority.[50]

Gilles's third and much longer poem, also of historical interest, the *De laudibus et virtutibus compositorum medicaminum*, is again a free adaptation of a famous Salernitan work, the *Glossae in Antidotarium* of Matthew Platearius. In this poem, Gilles addresses a revered master, Romualdus Guarna, not as a shade, but as a living person, establishing the fact that the *De laudibus* was begun sometime before 1181, the year of Romualdus's death.[51] Like all dispensatories this work underwent a continuous series of additions and revisions, with the result that the completed version of the poem probably did not appear until sometime after 1194, because the poem has a distinct reference in the last of the three books to the sack of Salerno.[52]

Gilles then wrote a new preface to the completed work describing the poem as *provectior aetas*, that is, of advanced age, or long delayed in writing. At this very period Gilles is referred to in highly laudatory terms by a namesake, Gilles de Paris, whose *Carolinus*, composed between 1191 and 1198, is, appropriately enough, another example of a didactic poem long in gestation. If Gilles did, in fact, return to Paris no earlier than 1194 to begin teaching, it is difficult to see how the reputation *celeberrimus in arte medendi* could possibly have been gained overnight.[53] Although himself a cleric, Gilles felt sufficiently secure under the protection of his royal patient, Philip Augustus, to defy ecclesiastical censure in producing his devastating *Hierapigra ad Prelatos*, a task which occupied the declining years of his life. He died about 1224.

The following are specific references to Maurus found in Gilles's writings:

At *De urinis* 343, Gilles pays respect to the *dogmata Mauri* acquired through a study of the latter's *Regulae Urinarum*. Again, the following passage

---

[46] Gilles identifies himself with the school established by Adam de Parvo Ponte (Vieillard, *Gilles*, pp. 440–441). L. Minio-Paluello, 1954, has finally resolved the confusion which formerly existed between Gilles's master and an Adam of Balsham (d. 1183) noting that the former was a highly regarded colleague of such luminaries as John of Salisbury, Peter Lombard, and Thierry of Chartres, and sat with them in judgment at the proceedings against Gilbert de la Porrée (p. 117). For Gilles's career at Salerno I follow the account of DeRenzi (*Storia Documentata*, pp. 301–309), except that he brings Gilles to Salerno in 1150, more than a decade too soon.

[47] See versus 346–348 of *De urinis* for a vitriolic attack on Montpellier and its doctrines. Gilles may well have been too ardent a controversialist, for Matthew Salomon and several other masters of Salerno had already found a happy home at Montpellier. (*Storia Documentata*, pp. 320–321; Bariety and Coury, 1963: p. 345.) I believe that after the fiasco at Montpellier Gilles—then in his mid-thirties—headed home to Paris rather than back to Salerno. Lawn, pp. 32, 69–72, has carefully reviewed the career and influence of this "apostle of Salerno to the north," but leaves us with an unexplained hiatus of two decades between Montpellier and 1194, at which time he would have Gilles begin his teaching at Paris. I do not believe that Gilles ever returned to Salerno (indeed the two early poems written explicitly for the benefit of his pupils already reflect nostalgia for alma mater), but began to teach at Paris between 1175 and 1180.

[48] The medical school established by Gilles may have been the one which still existed near the Petit-Pont in the middle of the thirteenth century (Minio-Paluello, p. 165).

[49] Neckham studied in Paris between 1175 and 1182, according to recent workers (Lawn, p. 72); Haskins (*Studies*, p. 360) identifies him as a "pillar of the school of the Petit-Pont." Seidler, p. 59, notes that Neckham later calls Paris a city where *medicina viget*, while a contemporary, Guy de Bazoches, who also studied at the Petit-Pont, alludes to the school as *fons doctrine salutaris*. I believe that these references, coupled with Neckham's unusual familiarity with the Salernitan Questions, as well as with the contents of the *Articella* and the recently recovered *Libri naturales* of Aristotle (Haskins, *Studies*, pp. 373–375) all suggest that Neckham had some unusually close association with a master of Salerno, such as he could readily have acquired within the orbit of Gilles de Corbeil. It is now thought that Neckham wrote his *De natura rerum* at St. Albans shortly after his return to England (*ca.* 1185) while the recollections of his

medical studies at Paris were still fresh. See our Commentary note 88.

[50] Talbot, pp. 48–50, also discusses the strangely opposing attitude toward Salerno of Neckham and his intimate friend, Alfred of Sareshel. Almost half of the scientific topics discussed by Neckham have some relationship to the Salernitan Questions.

[51] The reference is to *De laudibus* 1.140. When Gilles invokes the shades of his masters, Matthew Platearius (1.100-111) and Musandinus (1.100), there can be no doubt that these beloved masters are no longer alive. There is no indication of such regret in his request for the sponsorship of the living Romualdus.

[52] *De laudibus* 3. 508–511.

[53] *Aegidii Parisiensis Carolinus sive de Gestis Caroli Magni*, ed. M. J. B. Briel, in *Recueil des Historiens des Gaulles et de la France* (Paris, 1818) 17: pp. 288–301. In the presumably later works by Gilles, the *Liber de signis et symptomatibus aegritudinum*, the *Versus super Pronostica* (our note 107 below) and the *Hierapigra*, there are no references to Salerno.

tells us a good deal about events at Salerno immediately after Musandinus' death:

Spiritus [Musandini] exultat, et magni pectora Mauri
Tota replet; Maurus redimit damnumque rependit
Prima quod in Petro [Musandino] passa est et perdidit
    aetas
Qui tanquam manus humeris colloque gigantis
Desuper incumbens ipso fortasse tuetur
Longus, et summo superaddit culmina monti.
                                                    (*De laudibus* 1.94–99)

The great Musandinus is dead, but in Maurus he has been replaced by a not unworthy successor.

Elsewhere, Gilles emphasizes Maurus's role as protector of the school:

Suppleat et Petri (Musandini] Maurus mihi damna
    reformet
Pastor ovem, membrumque caput, famulumque patronus,
Doctor discipulum, noscat sua mater alumnum.
                                                    (*De laudibus* 1.107–109)

From additional verses, we learn that Maurus was an outstanding personality who achieved great success in the courtly and wealthy circles of Salerno.[54] His costly armamentarium included the famous *diamargariton*, which contained two varieties of crushed pearls in Falernian wine, as well as other preparations composed in part of amber, precious stones and gold. Gilles himself may have been of peasant stock and, at any rate, seems to have had a warm feeling for the needy. Perhaps Maurus, the "aulic physician," had too little time to spare for the Codrus-like patient, suffering from a "spasm of the purse," and Gilles chides his master none too gently:

An quia deficiunt species et aromata
Codrizant tua, Codre, salus, deiecta fatiscit
Corpora integritas, que te presentia Mauri
Splendida non recreat, multo spectabilis auro.[55]

MAURUS OF SALERNO:
LIFE AND INFLUENCE

The place and date of Maurus's birth are unknown,[56] but he was probably born of a noble family

about 1130 in a part of sourthern Italy where some Greek was still spoken.[57] He studied medicine at Salerno under Matthew Platearius and Peter Musandinus about 1150–1160, and became a leader of the circle of younger masters surrounding Musandinus. The latter died about 1165,[58] and after a brief interlude, Maurus assumed the honorary post of headmaster. By this period the Constantinian translations had been current at Salerno for well over half a century, and the Arabic texts were threatening to overwhelm the school's earlier writings and traditions. Because Maurus's own teachers had been men of a conservative stamp, he also made a valiant but vain attempt to sustain lagging interest in the older texts. The most obvious influence in his own work is that of Hippocrates, whose *Aphorisms* he must have studied

---

[54] Royal interference at Salerno was so strong that masters had little control over the standards and regulations affecting the teaching and practice of medicine (Bullough, pp. 49–51). H. Rashdall (1936: 1: p. 83) asserts that the *licentia medendi* was controlled by the court bureaucracy. Haskins (*Studies*, p. 250) suggests that the regulations of 1231 simply intensified bureaucratic control and acted as a hindrance to further academic development. For similar interference at Montpellier see A. Luchaire, p. 66.

[55] *De laudibus* 2.93, 99–102. Codrus, a penurious poet, contemporary with Juvenal, became a symbol of poverty. The entire section (verses 68–123) seems to be addressed to Maurus, and is at once a eulogy of sobriety and a denouncement of the excesses of the wealthy. In *De laudibus* 4.1446–1481, Gilles exhorts his students to assist the needy even by exacting contributions from the rich.

[56] Secondary sources include DeRenzi *Storia Documentata*, pp. 332–335; Steinschneider, "Maurus," *Virchows Archiv* **40** (1867): pp. 91–94, and *Die Hebraeischen Übersetzungen*, p. 810;

also F. Hartmann, *Die Literatur von Früh-und Hoch-Salerno* (Leipzig, 1919). St. Maurus had been a favorite disciple of St. Benedict at Subiaco and Monte Cassino, and his cult, particularly strong in Benedictine Campania, was often invoked, especially against rheumatic diseases. John, Maurus's father, is designated as *comes* in a legal document (*Storia Documentata*, p. li). In the *De laudibus* 1.121, Gilles addresses one cryptic line to Maurus: *Urso suum te concivem gaudebit adesse.* Why especially Urso? If the term "fellow-citizen" has any special significance, it may imply that Maurus, like Urso, originally came from Calabria (Creutz, *Urso*, p. 6). Maurus does praise the wines of Calabria as useful in the treatment of strangury and bladder stone (*CS* 4: p. 553). G. Augelluzzi, 1853: p. 18 calls Maurus and Urso natives of Salerno, but cites no evidence for this.

[57] During the tenth century, the counts of Salerno usually paid allegiance to the eastern emperor. Haskins (*Studies*, chap. 8) traces the survival of the Greek language in southern Italy. Merchants of Amalfi and Salerno continued an active interchange of goods with Byzantium, and Archbishop Alfanus (*d.* 1085), the translator of Nemesius, spent some time in the capital collecting Greek codices. Stephen of Pisa (1127) says: "In Sicily and at Salerno where students of such matters [medicine] are chiefly to be found, there are both Greeks and men familiar with Arabic" (Haskins, *Studies*, p. 133). The Norman court published edicts in Latin, Greek, and Arabic, according to need. It is not therefore surprising that Maurus should have acquired a very superficial acquaintance with Greek. He frequently uses Greek medical terms when Latin equivalents are available, and such usage may have been common practice rather than mere affectation. He does take a truly scholastic delight in supplying his students with a *derivatio nominis*, even though his explanation is, at times, more fanciful than accurate. Our own text supplies reasonable derivations for *leucoflegmantia, hyposarca, anasarca, hypostasis and nephilis*, but the three alternative explanations for *urina* are equally fanciful and incorrect (*CS* 4: p. 407), as is the association of *plegmio* and *pulmo* (our text 28.15). Of the two suggested derivations for *antrax* (our text 7.7–16), one is fanciful, the other is reasonably correct. Interestingly enough, he interchanges *phisis* and *natura* in the same paragraph (our text 16.17–20), and invariably uses *sintoma* in preference to the classical *symptoma*. But *oresinon* (our text 28:68) is a pure Greek word. Maurus's knowledge of Greek was weak, limited to a few technical terms, and may have been based on gloss collections: it is almost certain that he could not read the language even in a rudimentary sense.

[58] The date of Musandinus's death is critical for the entire problem of Gilles de Corbeil and his relationship to Salerno. It seems certain that Gilles knew Musandinus in the flesh, and probably saw Maurus succeed him. Because Musandinus was a pupil and successor of Bartholomaeus, who died about 1150, Musandinus may well have died about 1165 as DeRenzi thought (*Storia Documentata*, p. 317).

with constant care and devotion. For Maurus, Hippocrates cannot err, and any apparent discordance between authorities must result in a solution consistent with the doctrines of the Master.[59]

As the tide of Arabism continued to rise unrelentingly during Maurus's maturity, another powerful intellectual force was gradually making itself felt at Salerno. Haskins long ago noted the importance of the Salernitan medical community as a center for the attraction and diffusion of scientific knowledge,[60] but it remained for Birkenmajer to point out that Maurus and Urso were among the very first to benefit by the new Greek-to-Latin translations of Aristotle's *libri naturales*.[61] From the standpoint of medical progress, this initial contact with speculative philosophy proved not an unmixed blessing, because it served to divert younger physicians like Urso from the practical aspects of medicine to abstract theory. Maurus himself was probably too much of a traditionalist by temperament to be swept completely under the spell of the new logic, and his published writings reveal only a superficial familarity with the subtle distinctions, refinements, and syllogistic reasoning of mature scholasticism.[62]

We have already learned from Gilles that Maurus was a man of impressive personality and commanding presence, equally distinguished as teacher and practitioner. Maurus's intimate association with his wealthy and courtly patrons may have served to temper the petty interference to which the masters of the school were constantly being subjected. From the large number of his surviving works, we must assume that his career as a teacher was a long one, and he may well have retained the position of headmaster in 1194 when Salerno was sacked by the troops of Henry VI.[63] With this tragic event began the gradual decline of Salerno from its position as the leading medical center of Europe. Foreign students deserted the town for Montpellier and Paris, and the school never recovered completely from this blow.

That a lowering of standards of teaching did occur at this very period we learn from the *De laudibus*. Gilles, now in Paris, decries the sad state of affairs at his *alma mater*, where the ancient texts and customs have been discarded, and callow, poorly trained youths are being sent forth as masters.[64] It was also at this very period, about 1200, when Urso *philosophus* had taken over from Maurus as the leader of the medical community, that teaching aids, the so-called "Salernitan Questions," reached their fullest development. Maurus contributed, at most, only two questions to this list whereas Urso is credited with no fewer than ten.[65] The rise in popularity of such didactic aids to memory would thus seem to parallel a general deterioration of medical standards at Salerno. It is difficult to believe that the scholarly Maurus could have looked with satisfaction on such short-cuts to medicine.[66] Indeed, from this time onward the scholastic method which had originally proved so useful in the improvement of classroom

---

[59] For example, Maurus wrote a preface to the venerable *Antidotarium*, thus adding the prestige of his name to this classic of the school (*Storia Documentata*, p. 334), while Gilles deplores the neglect of the true Salernitan doctrines as expounded by Musandinus in favor of alien (= Arabic) writings filled with errors (Vieillard *Gilles*, pp. 171, 343), and vows to revive them in a more attractive and modern form. DeRenzi (*Storia Documentata*, p. 306) cites the writings of Matthew Platearius to sustain his contention that Salerno remained relatively free from *il vero Arabismo* until the second half of the twelfth century. The reverence shown to Hippocrates in our text (he is mentioned sixty-five times by name or as *auctor*) involves Maurus in spirited defense of the Master (see our text 12; 34.77–84 and 42). Only on one occasion does Maurus contradict the Master (see our text 40.77–89 and its commentary), and this difference may perfectly well involve a scribal error.

[60] Haskins *Renaissance*, p. 293.

[61] C. Dickson, 1934: pp. 121–122 and Schipperges, 1964, p. 64, are among those who hold this position. The latter believes that by 1170 Maurus was already familiar with Aristotle's *Physica* in the *vetera translatio* attributed to James of Venice (1128) and that he may have had access to the *Liber sufficientis* of Gundisalinus (1120–1140), in turn derived from Avicenna's *Kitab-as Sifa*. He further concludes (pp. 61, 67, and 153) that Maurus knew the Aristotelian *De caelo et mundo* and the *De generatione et corruptione* as well as the Avicennan *De actionibus et passionibus*, the two latter works in the translation of Henricus Aristippus of Catania (d. 1162). A. Birkenmajer, 1930: p. 5, and more recently Lawn, p. 180, have also noted the strong Aristotelian influence in Maurus's Commentary on the *Isagoge* of Johannitius, still unpublished. Birkenmajer shows considerable familiarity with the contents of B.N. lat. 18499, but fails to cite the library location. Evident in our own Commentary is the beginning of a didactic style, a tendency to over-elaboration, and an artificially diffuse system of explanation and argument. Through the *Pantegni* and the *Isagoge* Salerno had received all the elements of the scholastic method long before this valuable aid to instruction became available through the Toledan translations of Aristotle. However, in Maurus, although there is considerable prolixity, dry formalism, and overly ambitious attempts at etymology, there is none of the purely syllogistic approach, or the excessive subtlety which was to characterize the full-blown scholasticism of the thirteenth century.

[62] This statement may require modification when Maurus's commentary on Johannitius is published. It is interesting to note that the fame, power, and admiring friends offered by Maurus as inducements to prospective medical students (our text 2.7) harks back to the Hippocratic prognosticator as envisioned by Edelstein, p. 76, rather than to the austerities of Galen, who had been taught by this father "to stress modesty and forego the esteem of people" (Siegel, 1968: p. 7).

[63] In 1191 the ailing empress Constance, then under treatment by the physicians of Salerno, was briefly held as a hostage by Tancred, thus inspiring the emperor's wrath against the city, and providing an excuse for its wanton destruction three years later.

[64] For Gilles's adverse reaction to current developments at Salerno, see Vieillard, *Gilles*, pp. 198–199, 356–357, and *De laudibus* 3.564–577.

[65] Lawn, p. 203, notes that the popular question *solis calor* deriving from Seneca is discussed by Maurus, as is the possibility that fever may be induced by foods seasoned by pepper and garlic (B.N. lat. 18499 *Super Isagoge Ioanitii* 26v, 31).

[66] One of Maurus' complaints against the sectists is that they attempt to explain *totam artem sub brevibus capitulis* (*CS* 4: p. 515).

exposition was to be pushed to a degree where it was to become an actual hindrance to progress.[67]

Maurus lived on until 1214,[68] but long before then he may have relinquished his practice to his sons Matthew and John, both *magistri in phisica*.[69] His wife, Theodora, died in 1239, surviving Maurus by twenty-five years.[70]

The fame Maurus had acquired during a long lifetime persisted after his death. In the necrology of the Cathedral of San Matteo at Salerno, he is the only physician of the more than eighty listed who is honored by the title *optimus fisicus*;[71] one manuscript calls him *secundus Galienus Salernitanus*;[72] another work ends with *hoc opus a Mauro restat, pretiosus auro*, and a third asserts *inde cunctis Maurus mortalibus est venerandus*.[73] Rufinus includes Maurus among the wise men of Salerno and quotes him as an authority on several occasions, once indeed when there was *maxima diversitas inter sapientes*.[74] Maurus is one of only two *moderni* included in the library of a certain thirteenth-century Tuscan surgeon,[75] while the early fourteenth-century student at the Sorbonne could still consult the *De urinis* in the *magna libraria*.[76] Such eminent authorities as Gentile da Fuligno[77] and Lanfranco[78] quote him with respect. Steinschneider notes that Maurus was greatly admired by the Jewish physicians who translated his tracts on the urine, simple fevers, and phlebotomy, and that the Pseudo-Asaph called him "the learned teacher Mor,

the Christian from Salerno."[79] Birkenmajer[80] notes that Maurus's commentaries on the *Articella* were known and used by Raoul Longchamp (born *ca.* 1155), and that they served as a model for later commentators including Roland of Cremona. Vincent of Beauvais quotes him repeatedly in the *Speculum maius*.[81] Finally, through the poem *De urinis* of Gilles de Corbeil and its many commentators, the *dogmata Mauri* continued to exert some influence for several centuries.[82]

Maurus has been greatly admired by medical historians of the past century. Haeser, Puschmann, Diepgen, and especially Sudhoff regard him as the representative teacher and protagonist of the school of Salerno at the very apex of its property.[83] Many factors contributed to the eventual decline of Salerno as a center of medical education; the rivalry of Montpellier and Paris, the rise of the schools of northern Italy and the influence of nearby Naples all contributed to the inevitable result. Nevertheless, it may be fairly stated that at no time did Salerno enjoy greater fame and authority than during the three or four decades during which Maurus dominated the academic scene.

MAURUS: THE PRINTED WORKS[84]

Anatomia Mauri: Corner[85] and Sarton[86] identify this as the third Salernitan anatomical demonstration.

[67] Bayon, p. 205; Talbot, p. 44.

[68] Garufi, pp. 85, 216. Maurus died on February 24, 1214.

[69] For Matthew see Capparoni, p. 33, and for Matthew and John see A. Sinno, pp. 133–134. Matthew must have been a man of considerable distinction, a worthy son of a worthy father. He became personal physician and confidant to Tomasso da Montenegro, Justiciar to Frederic II. Son John, named after his paternal grandfather, was presumably author of the *Cure Magistri Johannis Mauri* (Codex Prague 2614, ff. 66v–67). R. Calvanico, p. 918 (120) mentions a surgeon named Matteo de Mauro, who practiced in Naples in the fourteenth century, and may well have been a late descendant. Indeed, a Matthew is listed as a grandson of Maurus's son John in the document cited in note 56 above.

[70] Capparoni, p. 43.

[71] The medical men listed in Garufi include such celebrities as Musandinus, Salernus, and Urso.

[72] Puccinotti, 2: p. xxviii.

[73] Sudhoff, *Die vierte Salernitaner Anatomie*, p. 35.

[74] L. Thorndike, *The Herbal of Rufinus* (Chicago 1946), pp. 17, 69, 317.

[75] Coturri, p. 79.

[76] Seidler, p. 59: the list is dated 1338. Maurus's *Practica* could still be studied in a fifteenth-century north Italian library, as noted by E. Lazzareschi, 1925: p. 123. His name also appears in the catalog of St. Augustine's Abbey, Cambridge, "drawn up about the end of the fifteenth century" (Cholmeley, pp. 115–116).

[77] Gentilis de Fulgineo, *Super Primaseu Quarti Canonis Avicennae* (Venice, 1514), pp. 41–42, 56, and see our note 101 below. Gentile fully recognizes the close relationship between the *De urinis* of Maurus and the verses of Gilles.

[78] Sarton, *Introduction* 2: p. 1080; Lanfranchi (d. 1306), "Father of French Surgery."

[79] Steinschneider, 1868: p. 94.

[80] Birkenmajer, pp. 5, 14. Raoul wrote a commentary on the *Anticlaudianus* of his master, Alain de Lisle.

[81] Creutz, 1938: p. 309, notes that Maurus is mentioned in books 28 and 31 of the *Speculum Naturale* and in books 12, 13, and 14 of the *Speculum Doctrinale*, thus making him the most frequently cited of the native Salernitan physicians.

[82] Sudhoff, 1929, pp. 129–135, elaborates on the continuing influences of Maurus's teachings, *via* the verses of Gilles, on medieval uroscopy. See also P. Diepgen's edition of the *Summa medicinalis* of Walter Agilinus, pp. 15, 24–27 and 31–35. H. E. Handerson, 1918: p. 41 epitomizes the chapter on dropsy of Gilbertus Anglicus (fl. 1250); obviously his comments are a direct paraphrase of the discussion in our text (15.1–30).

[83] Haeser, 1: p. 669; Pushmann *Handbuch* 1: p. 653; *Sudhoffs Archiv* 20 (1928): p. 55, and *Archeion* 14 (1932): p. 363; Pazzini, 1944: 1: p. 417, and Diepgen's edition cited in note 82 above.

[84] The following writings are attributed to Maurus of Salerno:
In print: (1) *Anatomia Mauri* (ed. Ploss; Corner; Sudhoff); (2) *De Flebotomia* (ed. Buerschaper); (3) *Regulae Urinarum* (ed. Kadner; *CS* 3: pp. 1–51, *CS* 4: pp. 400–412); (4) *Commentary on the Aphorisms of Hippocrates* (*CS* 4: pp. 513–557); Italian translation by Stroppiana and Minghetti (Rome, 1959); (5) *Commentary on the Prognostics of Hippocrates*, Latin text and English translation printed here for the first time; (6) *Pillulae Mauri* (*CS* 3: p. 51 and *Storia Documentata*, p. xlvi).
In manuscript: For a full description of the contents of B.N. lat. 18499, see pp. 33–34 above; *Commentary on the Prognostics of Hippocrates* (Vat. lat. 4477 ff. 37–48; B.N. lat. 7102, prologue only, with marginal glosses, f. 137); *Practica* (Stift Neukloster B.3 ff. 74–(55); *De Sterilitate* (BMsl 3124 ff. 331v–354); *De Febribus Compositis* ((BMsl 342 ff. 139v–145; *Regulae Medicinae* (Valicelliana B61). For a complete list of tracts on uroscopy attributed to Maurus see Thorndike and Kibre (1963) col. 394, 948, 1271, 1609.
Mentioned: *De medicina laxative* (Thorndike, *Rufinus*, p. 69);

It is briefer than the second, and less obviously derived from the *Pantegni*, but it cannot be claimed that Maurus demonstrates much originality in this work, and in fact many of his descriptions are merely rewordings of the preceding texts. Corner found no evidence of scholasticism in this presumably early work and identified the translation of Hippocrates used as the *antiqua translatio* attributed to Constantinus in the earliest printed texts. Although Maurus never mentions Constantinus in this tract, the inclusion of such Arabic terms as *meri, siphac, zirbum,* and *mirix* indicates the ultimate source of much of his information. Following Isaac, Maurus does not differentiate accurately between the nerves and tendons,[87] but he correctly equates the *panniculus ausungiae qui dicitur siphac* (peritoneum) with the *epigasunta hymenon*. Because these terms mean "fatty membrane" in Greek, Latin, and Arabic, it seems likely that some degree of familiarity with the technical vocabulary of all three languages was common in professional circles.[88] In his excellent description of the passage of blood from the liver to the *vena concava* and through the heart to the *adhortum*, Maurus follows closely his immediate predecessor, probably Bartholomaeus.[89] He also agrees that the Arabic *meri* refers only to the *os stomachi* and not to the entire *ysophagus*. Maurus prefers *ysmon* to *isthmus* and *oscheon* to *oxeum* or *scrotum*. The use of the term *ypochondria superiora* to describe the cavities above the diaphragm is perhaps unique to Maurus,[90] and is found again in our own text of the *Commentary on the Prognostics*.[91]

De Flebotomia: This small work shows Maurus at his best as wise clinician and teacher. Although he mentions Hippocrates, the *Megategni* of Galen, Alexander of Tralles, and Constantinus as authorities, there is evidence on every page of much original thought and judgment. On several occasions he refuses to bleed excessively as recommended by other authors, adding *nos autem timemus vulgi opinionem.*[92]

The *De flebotomia* became so popular that it eventually superseded the pseudo-Hippocratic *Epistola Flebotomiae* of unknown date which had long held the field.[93] Maurus gives explicit instructions as to the season, day, and hour best suited for the procedure, his opinion being based on the age, habits, and strength of the patient, and on the dominant humor. His theory of a diurnal variation of the humors seems to be original, and was widely accepted as authoritative.[94] In cases of cerebral abscess with phrenitis, Maurus recommends opening the venules of the nares by means of pig bristles; in bites of poisonous animals, blood should be let *per metacentesim*, that is, from the injured side, in order to protect the noble members. Throughout this work, Maurus displays a keen historical sense, weighing the opinions of the *antiqui* against the *moderni* before arriving at his own decision. At one point, he notes differences between the masters of Salerno and Montpellier in the classification of fevers.[95] On the negative side, we may point to the traditional avoidance of the new moon and the dog days for bleeding, and the application of animal dung to reduce swelling of the veins and nerves. The entire tone of the work is authoritative and guardedly optimistic, in marked contrast to the conservative and often depressing language which dominates the *Commentary on the Prognostics*. Maurus's reputation as an authority on phlebotomy remained very high during the Middle Ages, his work being consulted not only by the physician but by the veterinarian as well.[96]

Regulae Urinarum: The high esteem in which Maurus's name was held throughout the Middle Ages can be traced, in large part, directly to this, his most influential single work, one which has often been termed the best medieval tract on uroscopy.[97]

Liber serbortaneum (?) (Coturri, p. 79); *Cura nymphomaniae* (Puccinotti, 2, p 1: p. xxviii); *De Febribus Simplicis* (Steinschneider, *Hebraische Übersetzungen*, p. 810). The *Antidotarium Mauri* (*Storia Documentata*, p. 306) is the ancient *Antidotarium* with a new preface by Maurus.

[85] Corner, *Anatomical Texts*, p. 29.

[86] Sarton, *Introduction* 2: p. 436.

[87] Ploss, p. 7: *sex nervi sive lacerti.*

[88] Ploss, p. 8. For the Arabic terms found in Maurus, see Adolf Fonahn, *Arabic and Latin Anatomical Terminology* (Christiana, 1922).

[89] Ploss, p. 8; Sudhoff, *Codex Fritz Paneth*, p. 29.

[90] Ploss, p. 8.

[91] Our text, chapter 10.

[92] Buerschaper based his 1919 text on two manuscripts (Dresden Db 91, 62r–63r, and Brussels 14324–14343, 242ff.), both actually ascribed to Maurus; the latter can now be identified with two additional manuscripts (New College, Oxford 1135 and Laurentian codex 33, Pluteus 73). Henry of Wendover may have been the translator of this popular work, but could not have been the original author as Talbot, p. 63 suggests. Thorndike-Kibre

(col. 1086) lists seven other versions of the text, variously ascribed or anonymous. Mention of the *Megategni* of Galen (Buerschaper, p. 8), one of the Constantinian translations, indicates that this longer work, as well as the *Ars Parva* or *Tegni*, was studied at Salerno.

[93] The *Epistola Flebotomiae* is closely related to a tract, *De Minutione Sanguinis sive De Phlebotomia*, long attributed to Bede (J. F. Payne, 1904: pp. 16–19), but denied by W. Sharpe, 1955–1956: pp. 62–87. See also Meyer-Steinegg and Sudhoff, 1956: p. 186. Maurus's work was copied freely by other Salernitans (Buerschaper, pp. 28–29).

[94] See pp. above.

[95] Buerschaper, pp. 15–16. "Nota quod huius modi febres, quae comitantur huiusmodi apostemata, dicuntur effimer[ae] secundum Salernitanos secundum magistros Montis Pessuli quaedam dicuntur putrid[a]e." For the rivalry which already existed between the two schools during Maurus's lifetime, see the account of a Bartholomaeus Ultramontanus who, having failed at Salerno, departed in high dudgeon for Montpellier (Sudhoff, *Salerno, Montpellier und Paris*, p. 53).

[96] Luigi Barbieri, ed., *Lorenzo Rusio: La Mascalcia* (Bologna, 1867); 1: p. 82: *Magister Maurus dixit, quod equus, ut praeservaretur a diversis et variis infermitatibus, debet ad minus ter in anno minui.* There is another reference to Maurus at p. 320. Rusio (fl. 1288) was a pioneer in the revival of the veterinary art.

[97] Pazzini, 1944: 1: p. 481, finds agreement between the

The indebtedness to Theophilus, on whose *Urinae* Maurus had already written (or was to write) a commentary and to the *De urinis* of Isaac Judaeus is obvious, but the *Regulae* is in no sense a mere compendium, and in clarity of expression and arrangement, marked a distinct advance over its predecessors. Self-confidence and conviction pervade this obviously mature work, nor does Maurus hesitate to criticize his two authorities, noting that in their definition of the *urine, neutrum tamen verum est*.[98] Maurus mentions Constantinus at least five times in the DeRenzi text, and the strong scholastic bent, already noted by Sudhoff, merely indicates that even the conservative Maurus could no longer resist the trend to formalism, speculation, and over-elaboration which was soon to overwhelm the Salernitan writings.

Although diagnosis *per urinam* is the ostensible purpose of the *Regulae*, Maurus digresses to expound his views on a wide variety of related topics. The humoral theory, physiology of digestion, classification of fevers, mental derangements, jaundice, and diabetes are but a few of the subjects considered in this important work. Gilles de Corbeil freely acknowledges that his own verses were inspired by the teachings of his Salernitan masters, and, as has been noted previously, it was through his popular poem, *De urinis*, that the *dogmata Mauri* were to continue to exert some influence for at least three centuries. The wide acceptance of the *Regulae* as a standard work is indicated by the large number of manuscripts identifying Maurus as the author, and by an even larger number of anonymous tracts deriving directly or indirectly from the original.[99]

Commentary on the Aphorisms: The *Aphorisms* of Hippocrates is the work which Maurus admired above all others, and to which he most often refers in his own writings. As we have noted, Corner demonstrated that Maurus used the Constantinian translation of the *Aphorisms* with Galen's commentary in preparing his own glosses. He might also have known the earlier translation with Oribasius's commentary. Salerno had long cherished this famous work, and Talbot considers Copho's *Ars Medendi* or *Practica* as little more than a commentary on the

Aphorisms.[100] In this commentary, Maurus elaborates his most famous theory that of the diurnal variations of the humors, in which he assigns a period of six hours to each of the four humors:

	Atmosphere	Dominant Humor
3 P.M.–9 P.M.	Warm and Dry	Bile
9 P.M.–3 A.M.	Cold and Dry	Black Bile
3 A.M.–9 A.M.	Cold and Humid	Phlegm
9 A.M.–3 P.M.	Warm and Humid	Blood

This *orarium* was consulted to determine the time best suited for administering purges and other medications as well as for bloodletting. It was considered authoritative by no less a master than Gentile da Foligno,[101] and is cited by Alexander Neckham as well as by Bartholomew the Englishman.[102] DeRenzi selected this renowned work as the single most typical example of Salernitan learning in anatomy, physiology, diagnosis, and therapy, and provided a very thorough analysis of the text.[103]

THE PROGNOSTICS OF HIPPOCRATES

Recent studies tend to minimize the close relationship formerly thought to exist between the *Prognostica*, the *Prorrhetica*, and the *Coacae Praenotiones*, and the *Prognostica* is now more than ever regarded as one of the few pure expressions of authentic Hippocratic thought.[104] Close association of this text with the more popular *Aphorisms* began in ancient times, and the translation of both works by Hunain-ibn-Ishaq in the ninth century inspired their wide dissemination throughout the Arab world.

As for the West, it has long been known that certain minor elements of the Hippocratic corpus were already being read in Latin at the Vivarium of Cassiodorus. Latin translations of the *Aphorisms*

---

anatomical knowledge of the *Regulae* and the *Anatomia*, and notes that Maurus distinguishes four zones in the urine glass, corresponding to the principal organs of the body:

Circulus.....................Brain and organs of animation
Superfluitas................Heart and lungs
Substantia..................Liver and organs of nutrition
Fundus.....................Kidneys and testes

[98] Kadner 4. In DeRenzi's version (*CS* 3: p. 2) Maurus terms Isaac's definition of urine *quidam erroneam*.

[99] Aside from the three printed texts, there are numerous manuscript versions (Thorndike-Kibre, cols. 394, 948, 1271). Gilles, while freely admitting his indebtedness to Maurus, denounces the plagiarists of his own work (Vieillard, *Gilles*, pp. 189–190), yet he never acknowledges the debt owed by the Salernitan uroscopists to the Arabs. For a discussion of Maurus's views on fever, see W. W. Anschutz, 1919: p. 30.

[100] Corner *Anatomical Texts*, p. 25; Pazzini confirms Maurus's familiarity with Galen's commentary (Stroppiana-Minghetti, pp. 11–17); see also Talbot, pp. 40–41. Beccaria, pp. 461–462, lists five manuscripts of the *Aphorisms*, one in Beneventan script dating to the eighth century, and thirteen with the Oribasius commentary.

[101] DeRenzi (*CS* 4: pp. 520–522, and *Storia Documentata*, p. 334) provides the references to Gentile. The latter considers Maurus the originator of this theory, and expresses admiration for the explanation of the mechanism whereby the body transfers destructive matter (as in squinantia) from noble to ignoble parts. This theory is mentioned at least six times in our own text, which Gentile may well have known.

[102] Lawn, p. 194, quotes Bartholomew: *In aurora autem humor sanguinis principaliter dominatur*.

[103] DeRenzi, *Storia Documentata*, pp. 365–370. In those instances where the *Commentary on the Aphorisms* expands upon topics briefly noted in the *Commentary on the Prognostics*, we refer to appropriate sections of the printed text (*CS* 4: pp. 513–557).

[104] Compare the divergent opinions of Francis Adams, 1849: 1: p. 190, and L. Edelstein, 1967: pp. 71–72. For the transmission of the *Prognostics*, see Beccaria, 1959: p. 9. Sigerist, 1961: 2: p. 266, also inclined "to the belief that the Corpus Hippocraticum does contain books written by the master himself."

and *Prognostics* arrived in Byzantine Italy at about the same time (*ca.* sixth century), but through the latinized version of Oribasius's commentary on the *Aphorisms*, this work gained a much wider distribution than the *Prognostics*. Of the thirteen pre-Constantinian manuscripts of Oribasius listed by Beccaria, two are in the Beneventan script. On the other hand, the two manuscripts of the *Prognostics* (second half of the ninth century) which have survived are both from the north (St. Gall, Milan) and would seem to have no direct relationship with Salerno.[105] As we have seen, unlike the *Aphorisms*, the *Prognostics* did not enter into the composition of the so-called *Summa* of the ninth century. It would thus seem likely that, although the *Aphorisms* had long been studied at Salerno, the complete text of the *Prognostics* did not become freely available until early in the twelfth century. And even though earlier commentaries on this work by Bartholomaeus and Musandinus are now known to exist, Maurus still approaches the less familiar text with an unusual degree of reverence.[106] Our *Commentary on the Prognostics* was obviously completed after the similar work on the

---

[105] 95.25, 108.16

[106] Kuehlewein devoted two articles to a study of medieval texts of the *Prognostics* (1884 and 1890), and in the latter published a ninth-century Latin translation from codex Ambrosianus G. 108 Inf., noting a very strong affinity with Caelius Aurelianus. Sigerist later (1930) published a fragment from St. Gall, cod. 44, also of the ninth century, which he considered somewhat later, written in a more vulgar Latin and less slavish than the Ambrosian text. Beccaria, pp. 288, 364, assigns both extant versions to the second half of the ninth century. A comparison of the two earlier versions with the text used by Maurus is useful:

St. Gall 44	Ambrosianus G.108 Inf.	Parisinus 18499
Dentes autem stridere in febre, quibus non est consuetudo a pueritia, et insano et mortale.	Dentes autem stridere in febre, cui solitum non est a pueritia, insaniae signum et mortale valde.	Frendere dentibus in febribus praeter solitum, nec a puero, mortem vel maniam significat.

The pseudo-Hippocratic *Capsula Eburnea*, written originally in Greek, had been translated into Latin by the sixth century, and appeared somewhat later in Syriac, Hebrew, Arabic, and Persian. This immensely popular tract known under various titles was aimed primarily at laymen rather than physicians, but contained much material derived from the Hippocratic *Prognostics*, including the *signa mortis* or *signa mortifera* (see Sigerist, 1958: p. 142; Sudhoff, 1916: pp. 79–116, and Kibre, 1945: pp. 387–389, 391–393).

The text of the translation of the *Prognostics* used by Maurus is closely related to that attributed to Constantinus in the two earliest incunabula of the *Articella* (Padua? 1476?, Venice 1483). However there are numerous *corrigenda* in spelling, grammar and wording which indicate a scrupulous revision and editing of the presumably more primitive text found in our manuscript. The Padua edition does not name the translator of Galen's commentary; the editor of the Venice edition (unnumbered page preceding p. 1) attributes this Latin translation to the hand of Gerard of Cremona. Because Gerard's translations had no influence on twelfth century Salerno, this would seem to strengthen the probability that Maurus did not have access to a twelfth century translation of Galen's *Commentary on the Prognostics*.

Aphorisms, but whereas the latter work is frequently named by Maurus in his other writings, I have thus far found only one direct reference to the Hippocratic *Prognostics*, and this may indicate that Maurus's glosses for this work were prepared rather late in life.[107] The *Prognostics* rejoin the *Aphorisms* in the earliest known versions of the *Articella*. Kristeller has described the process whereby various texts were added in the gradual development of this famous collection.[108]

The *Prognostics* of Hippocrates is concerned almost exclusively with acute febrile diseases which run a relatively short fulminating course, and which are not infrequently fatal. Temkin agrees with Littré that the Greek term *prognosis* had a much wider connotation than our present-day *semeiology*, and that the *Prognostics* contain much material which would now be classified as special pathology. Before preparing his prognostic statement, the Greek physician took into account not only the information supplied by relations as to the patient's former habits and appearance, but also such data as he could obtain by direct observation or through a study of the pulse and urine. Armed with the results of his thorough investigation, the physician finally delivered his authoritative prediction to the assembled family. Little wonder that the prognosis of such an exalted person seemed to be endowed with an almost oracular quality.[109]

Quite naturally, the tendency of the *Prognostics* is to generalize—to stress the universality of all symptoms common to acute febrile illnesses rather than the specific signs, good or bad, which may be observed in any individual disease. At a time when treatment was of limited and uncertain value, the prognosis had of necessity to be guarded, because the physician could often do little more than weigh the patient's resources and assess his ability to resist the disease.

---

[107] In the *Regulae Urinarum* (*CS* 3: p. 36), Maurus states: "Quod videtur innuere Ypocras in pronostica dicens 'Iuvenes qui sunt in hac passione magis depereunt. Veteres vero peripleumonie magis depereunt collectione." This agrees closely, but not verbatim with our text (37.12–30). Maurus may have been quoting from memory.

Thorndike-Kibre (col. 204) lists only one manuscript of the *Dicta super prognostica* attributed to Bartholomaeus, but no fewer than five manuscripts of glosses on the *Prognostica* by Musandinus (cols. 1277, 1619). There is also a twelfth-century *Glose super Pronostica Ypocratis* at Chartres (171, ff. 41–49) listed by Thorndike-Kibre (col. 850). If, as I believe, the verses by a hitherto unidentified Aegidius *Super Hippocratis Pronostica* (Edinburgh University Library MS 169 97v–106v) are actually by our Gilles, this would confirm the familiarity of Salerno with contents of the *Prognostics*.

[108] 1945: pp. 157–158; *Nuove Fonti*, pp. 62–63 *et passim*.

[109] For an elaboration of the subject of prognosis, see the studies of O. Temkin, 1928: pp. 36–39; W. H. S. Jones, *Hippocrates*, 2 (1923): pp. v–xxiii and Edelstein, 1967: pp. 65–85. The latter is alone in deprecating the scientific quality of the *Prognostics*. He finds little evidence of a logical theory of disease, but rather a tendency to dogmatic theorizing and rigid uniformity which he considers not characteristic of the Hippocratic writings.

The entire tone of the *Prognostics* is one of unrelieved pessimism, with emphasis on the inexorable advance of disease and the physician's professional futility. As will be seen, Maurus's own glosses do little to alter the Hippocratic mood.

ANALYSIS OF MAURUS'S COMMENTARY ON THE PROGNOSTICS OF HIPPOCRATES

Maurus's *Commentary* is a typical example of the class of *reportata*, in which the master's glosses adhere to each word or line of a classical text. In our brief analysis, emphasis is placed on Maurus's original interpretations, and the numbers refer to the number of the capitulum in the manuscript.

Prologue. 1. Maurus pays tribute to Hippocrates's brilliance and considers the origin, purpose, and plan of the *Prognostics*. He stresses the importance of the number three in describing the nature of matter, the body's active forces, and the signs of disease, the latter of which are derived from examination of the body's form, functions, and excretions. Maurus denounces empiric and methodist physicians, praises logical physicians, and traces the progression of medicine from practice to theory and philosophy. Prognostic signs excel all others in importance.

2. After extolling medicine's nobility as a profession, Maurus enters upon a philosophical discussion of health and the physician. He suggests means to win the patient's confidence, insisting that to avoid criticism, the physician must take a careful history and perform a thorough examination before making his prognosis which, in all cases, should be guarded. The causes of illness are natural or accidental; astronomy may be a useful tool in judging the nature and prognosis of an illness. The physician should abandon heroic treatment of a patient obviously moribund, but must spare no effect to make the dying man as comfortable as possible.

Section One. 3. The *Prognostics* is primarily concerned with acute, often fulminating, diseases and the first section is devoted to those diseases related to the animal forces, concentrated in the brain. Maurus quotes the nine favorable and unfavorable signs as outlined by Constantinus, but notes that a physician who has thoroughly examined a patient should not be censored if he incorrectly promises a return to health. The triad determining an object's appearance is Maker, substance, and form. The face has particular importance in prognosis because the five senses are located there. In reviewing the Hippocratic facies, Maurus adds his own notes on color, temperature, appearance of eyes, nose, and temples. He elaborates on the eyes: these are examined for protrusion, difference in size, bloody discoloration, discharge, mobility, and disposition during sleep. Maurus supplies a theory of vision, observing the close connection of the eye and brain. Impairment of sleep, elimination, and appetite are unfavorable signs.

4. The patient's posture in bed is elaborately considered: lying on the right side is best, but any position customarily adopted during health must be considered satisfactory. Excessive rigidity, slumping to the foot of the bed, carpholalgia, and irrational movements are dangerous signs. Grinding of teeth in children with fever is not too significant, but in adults, it may signify mental disease. Lying prone may indicate an abdominal abscess, lying supine, interference with respiration.

5. Maurus elaborates on posture in bed when the patient is so weakened that his death is near, when the pain of an abdominal abscess is relieved by compression of muscles in the prone position, and when a patient with pneumonia tries to raise himself in delirium, gasping for breath. Pus from pneumonia may lead to an inflammation of the brain.

6. Maurus returns to teeth grinding, voluntary or involuntary, citing pungent fumes, depletion of the nerves leading to the jaws and impaired digestion as primary causes of such involuntary activity. Grinding of the teeth may portend madness or death.

7. Maurus begins a discussion of abscesses, describing the various colors of abscesses derived from the four humors. Those which develop without fever are evacuated naturally, purulent matter which arises from a harmful humor is often transported from an ignoble to a noble organ, causing death. An ulcer which exists before the onset of a disease is less dangerous than one which develops during the course of an illness.

8. Movements of the hands have prognostic value in pneumonia with high fever, in abscesses, and in phrenitis accompanied by severe head pain. Picking at the walls and at the bedclothes may have ominous significance.

9. The mechanism of respiration is described and the interrelation of increased cardiac and respiratory activity is noted. Deep interrupted respiration may produce temporary loss of consciousness. If the exhaled air becomes cold, this is a fatal sign.

10. Maurus describes the four bodily excretions: sputum, feces, urine, and sweat, and discusses their origin and usefulness in prognosis. Sweat which is generalized, not excessive, and timely is a valuable sign; localized sweats of fetid odor and insipid taste or cold sweats which persist indefinitely weaken the patient and are of bad omen.

11. Maurus describes the four hypochondria and their contents. These cavities are frequent sites of abscess formation. It is a good sign if the two lower hypochondria are soft and equal; inequality with pulsation raises the suspicion of an abscess. A right-sided abdominal abscess is more to be feared, but an abscess in the upper left where the heart is located is

the most dangerous of all. Head pain and impaired vision suggest brain abscess. In such cases, nosebleed is to be hoped for to effect drainage.

12. Maurus describes the apparent differences between Hippocrates and Johannitius on the subject of sanguine abscesses. In general, abdominal abscesses are resolved by conversion into sanies or by a free flow of blood, the first method being preferable. Abscesses vary in shape, size, firmness, and duration; those below the umbilicus are less dangerous because of better drainage.

13–14. The abscess of black bile is the most persistent, often lasting sixty days. Abscesses pointing outward are readily evacuated; those absorbed internally without reaching the surface are not too dangerous, but those opening externally with a concealed inner portion are of bad prognosis, indicating weakness of natural heat and often end in a fistula. Indeed, it is better if no external opening develops. Only pus which is white in color, uniform in consistency, and free of evil odor may be considered to have a favorable connotation.

Section Two. 15. Hippocrates considers malfunctions related to the natural forces of the body, concentrated in the liver. Dropsy is the most important of these, and Maurus reviews the definition, causes and varieties of this condition, adding notes on etymology and pathology. Excessive strength of the expulsive virtue with opening of the pores may cause asthma. Each part of the body has a prefixed purpose and function which no other part can assume. Dropsy, although usually associated with liver dysfunction, may also arise from disorders of the intestinal tract, obstruction of the spleen, and respiratory tract involvement. Curable varieties of dropsy are leukoflegmantia and anasarca (hyposarca) because contraries may be cured by contraries; tympanites and ascites are more difficult to cure. Dropsy in acute fevers is particularly dangerous because no medication is effective. Persistent non-productive cough and swelling of the feet are of evil omen.

16. Dropsy may also arise from defect of the kidneys and from superfluities of the intestines which cannot be eliminated. If the abdomen is overheated while the head and extremities are cold, this is a dangerous sign. The diagnostic importance of discoloration of the nailbeds is considered at considerable length, but the color of the nails must be considered with additional signs before making a prognosis.

18. Maurus discusses the importance of the genitalia in prognosis: smallness of the penis may be due to loss of spirit or to an abscess; retraction of the testes may be caused by inanition, disturbance of the nerves, loss of humidity, or abscess formation. All these are dangerous signs.

19. Maurus turns from signs derived from the body's form to those derived from its activities. He then discusses the natural powers of the body and

shows how sleep arises when the visual spirit becomes inactivated and no longer reaches the eyes. Sleep is considered at length as to quantity, quality, and the period when it occurs. False sleep may be due to opium, phrenitis, or exhaustion following severe pain.

20–23. Maurus goes into a lengthy discussion of the intestinal superfluity or stool, stressing the importance of proper elimination. He describes various varieties of fecal discharge, discussing color, consistency, odor, and quantity in relation to food ingested. Passage of round worms is a desirable indication of strength of natural heat, and Maurus discusses the shapes of worms, indicating the varieties of phlegmatic humor involved in their production. The diagnostic value of the color of the fecal matter is again considered at length, as well as the origin and significance of flatulence. Excessive flatulence may result in swelling of the feet.

24–26. Maurus next provides a detailed discussion of urine, the superfluity of the second digestion. First he describes the physiology of digestion, including the roles of the stomach and liver, relating the quality of the urinary sediment to the effectiveness of digestion. Urinary sediments are considered as to color, uniformity, position in the urine-glass, and consistency. An excess of blood in the urine is undesirable, although not a fatal sign, and a coarse, scaly sediment implies a local bladder involvement. The various terms used in describing sediment in the zones of the urine-glass are mentioned. Of all colors, black is the most ominous whereas a uniformly white sediment indicates satisfactory completion of the third digestion. Urine with fatty particles in adults, and watery urine in children, are of the most serious importance.

27. Vomit is analyzed as to quantity, color, odor, consistency, and significance.

28. Sputum (or phlegm) may originate in the brain, stomach, or lungs. Maurus discusses sputum as to quantity, color, consistency, and odor. He distinguishes pleurisy from pneumonia, noting that reddish sputum at the beginning of pneumonia is characteristic and not dangerous unless continued after the seventh day. Prolonged hemorrhage from the lung or blackish expectoration are frequently of fatal significance.

29. Sneezing in catarrhal conditions is a bad sign, but when it occurs spontaneously, it is useful in clearing the brain. Labored expectoration without relief of pain is ominous, but Maurus warns against too hasty a prognosis in such cases, noting individual variations and the return of favorable signs.

30. Maurus returns to a discussion of abscesses, noting that the sanguine, phlegmatic, bilious, and atrabilious rupture in that order. He emphasizes the importance of determining the precise onset of chills and fever and the location of the abscess. He then

describes the symptoms of unresolved pneumonia: intermittent bouts of unproductive cough, persistent fever, loss of appetite, rapid respiration, and multiple secondary abscesses in the lower extremities. He notes the dramatic change for the better when the abscess breaks, but warns against a reaccumulation with recurrence of fever and renewal of symptoms.

31–32. Abscesses of the ears secondary to pneumonia are acute and often fatal in youths, but in the aged lead to chronic suppuration. Youths are more apt to be attacked by pleurisy, the aged by pneumonia, which is often terminal. Secondary infections may appear in the lower extremities.

33. Abscesses may also arise in the kidneys and bladder, the latter organ remaining free of pain unless the bilious humor is involved in the process. An abdominal abscess may thus compress the rectum and so interfere with the bladder. Because of the excessive humidity of the genitals, abscesses do not form there.

Section Three. 34. Maurus discusses favorable symptoms in that group of diseases which terminate by crisis, discoursing on critical days, the universality of the number twenty, and explains how to count by incomplete days in estimating the termination of fevers and abscesses.

35. He goes on to explain the delay in the remission of fevers in those obscure cases in which prognostic signs are not clear. He describes three- and four-day cycles and again warns that favorable signs may change at the peak of an illness.

36. He reviews conditions characterized by severe head pains, some of which are associated with fever, others with nasal hemorrhages. The latter is more apt to occur in the young, while older people develop secondary abscesses at some distance from the brain.

37. Ear involvement in youths with fever often leads to delirium and death. In the aged, there is more apt to be a continuuous discharge of pus from the ears, but youths die before pus can develop.

38–39. A variety of abscesses of the throat are defined and classified as to location, pathology, severity, chances of recovery, and forms of treatment.

40. The uvula is described and its function outlined. Principal complications of abscess of the uvula include suffocation, empyema, and phthisis. Before incising a uvular abscess, the patient should be thoroughly depleted by purgation.

41. Maurus considers fevers accompanied by paroxysms, the humors involved and the season of the year in which such paroxysms are apt to occur.

42. He continues a discussion of seasonal variation which has an influence on abscesses in general, and the manner whereby the various kinds of abscesses terminate. He includes the various classes of fevers, including intermittent fevers, which terminate by early or late crisis, vomiting, or nosebleed.

43. Maurus discusses convulsions in children and young people, the cause being extension and contraction of the nerves through repletion, inanition, or cold. High fever and constipation alone can produce convulsions in children younger than seven. In older youths, convulsions are usually associated with delirium.

44. In conclusion, Maurus follows Hippocrates in urging the physician to observe his patient closely as well as the signs which may be elicited from the excretions. He must also familiarize himself with epidemic and seasonal diseases frequently observed in the climate which prevails where he practices. Only by remaining faithful to the doctrines of Hippocrates will he avoid falling victim to the false teachings of pseudo-physicians.

THE MANUSCRIPT

History: Sanderus mentions a list of the manuscripts in the possession of the monastery of St. Martin at Tournai.[110] Our manuscript was sold in 1823, after the death of the Abbé Huré, and passed into the collection of the Parisian scholar, Arthur Dinaux. It appeared as item #813 of the Dinaux sale catalog, and as item #5894 at the actual sale, 2 December, 1864. Daremberg was the first to notice its acquisition by the Imperial Library in Paris.[111] Delisle describes the manuscript on several occasions,[112] and in more recent times, it has been cited by Corner,[113] Birkenmajer,[114] and Sudhoff.[115] In 1928 the latter first listed its contents and noted the scholastic tone of the commentaries; several years later, he returned to his "discovery" to emphasize its great importance and to urge full publication.[116] Kristeller revived interest in the manuscript,[116] and in 1950, drew the present writer's attention to Maurus's *Commentary on the Prognostics.*

Description: Bibliothèque Nationale MS latinus 18499. Manuscript on vellum, 209 leaves with a preliminary leaf A; end leaves from a fifteenth-century manuscript; sixteenth-century calf binding in good condition; some slight worming in early leaves. French thirteenth-century (Thorndike, personal communication, "northern France, not Italian"). Preliminary leaf A: *Nou. acq. lat* 79 and R. C. 5894.

[110] Antonius Sanderus, Bibliotheca Belgica Manuscripta (Insulis 1641–1644) part 1: p. 32, item G.25 *Catalogus alter MSS. librorum (Ecclesiae S. Martin Tornacensis) in pergameno.*

[111] C. Daremberg, *La Médicine, Histoire et Doctrines* (Paris, 1865), p. 461.

[112] Léopold Delisle, *Le Cabinet des manuscripts de la Bibliothèque Impériale* (Paris, 1868) 1: pp. 306–307; also *Bibliothèque de l'École des Chartes* (Paris, 1871) 31: pp. (463), 539; and *Inventaire des manuscrits de Notre-Dame et d'autre Fonds conservées a la Bibliothèque Nationale* (Paris, 1874), p. 99.

[113] Corner, *Anatomical Texts*, p. 26.

[114] Birkenmajer (see note 61 above) discusses at some length the philosophic content of Maurus's Commentary on the *Isagoge* of Johannitius, as does Lawn, pp. 27, 180, 203.

[115] Sudhoff, 1928: p. 55; 1932: p. 363.

[116] Kristeller, 1945: p. 158.

At the top of lr: *MAURUS SUPER YSAGOGAS.*
The text is divided into two columns; rubrication in
red and blue at the beginning of each text; the
lemmata are underlined in red; bizarre illustrations
on several pages.

TEXTS

1. Johannitius, Iasagoge: Incipit *Cum quelibet doc-
trinalis scientia humane utilitati,* explicit *et per accidens
existunt ideo ultimus modus est discretio boni vel mali
explicunt* (1rA–55rB).
2. Hippocrates, Aphorisms: Incipit *Cum omne corpus
animatum vel inanimatum,* explicit *a perturbationibus
ventus incepit et in fame librum suum terminavit
expliciunt glosule* (55vA–122vB).
3. Hippocrates, Prognostics: Incipit *Pronosticorum
Ippocratis fulgor inextricabilis arcam mentis,* explicit
*id est earum determinationis noticiam per mean, O
medice, doctrinam habebis* (123rA–144vB).
4. Theophilus, De urinis: Incipit *Quoniam ex tribus
tota humani corpora compago consistit,* explicit *et de
urinarum quidem disciplina et secundum genera et
secundum species et differentiae convenienter exposuimus
expliciunt glosule urinarum* (145rA–164rB).
5. Philaretus, De pulsibus: Incipit *Tocius humani
corporis machina triplicis participatione qualitatis,*
explicit *sed contrariis dicitur incidens nam incidens
et decidens sunt contrarii expliciunt glosule* (164vA–
171vB).
6. Galen, Tegni [Ars Parva]: Incipit *Ad omnem
artem ingressuri philosophantium,* explicit *Ipse enim
librorum suorum numero ponit et de quibus in unoquoque
agat manifeste dicit expliciunt glosule Tegni secundum
Maurum* (172rA–209rB).

CONCLUSION

There seems to be general agreement that Maurus
was a person of considerable ability, the "legislatore
della Scuola," who united in himself the qualities of
authority and leadership required to bring Salerno
to its highest peak of scholastic achievement. Maurus
prided himself on being a logical physician, one who
did not hesitate to oppose the *opinionem vulgi.* Conservative by nature and training, and ever mindful
of his position in the community, Maurus was nevertheless anxious to remain *au courant* with recent
developments in philosophy and science, especially
in so far as these might assist him in his professional
tasks. Although he follows the earlier scheme of
Bartholomaeus-Musandinus in relating theoretical
medicine to philosophy, I have found no evidence in
his published writings that he significantly disregards
natural phenomena or neglects the practical aspects
of the medical care of the patient. On the contrary,
he inveighs against vague and dogmatic generaliza-
tions, insisting on the equal importance of the
particularia with the *universalia.* Even his definition

of the subject confirms this view: *Medicine est scientia
que agit de hiis que ad usum et utilitatem humani
corporis sunt accomodata.*[117] He readily admits that
experience may be misleading at times, but insists
that when used with *rata ratio,* it offers the physician
the safest route to success.

Maurus is in the true Hippocratic tradition when
he recognizes that the physician is simply *naturae
minister,* and that *summa medicina est abstinentia.*
Certainly there can be no firmer denial of empiricism
than his remarkable statement, *si enim causam
ygnorat quomodo curat, et si forte aliquis ab eo curatus
evaserit, non erit sui muneris sed fortune.*[118] Yet
Maurus was obviously a man of his time, ambitious
for wealth and fame. If Gilles's assessment is valid,
Maurus may have been one of the Salernitan physicians castigated by John of Salisbury: "They put
into practice only two aphorisms: 'Do not labor where
there is poverty' and 'Take as much as you can as
long as the patient is sick.'"[119] It is true that in the
work published here—one which must represent a
mature distillation of the master's thought—there is
a definite tendency to elaboration and redundancy
which was to characterize thirteenth-century scholas-
icism. But while Maurus may have been eager to
demonstrate to his students an easy familiarity with
Aristotelian logic and terminology, these novelties
seem to have been poorly understood by him, and
aside from their usefulness as teaching aids, bear only
a superficial relevance to the subject matter of our
very practical text. Maurus may have been shrewd
and worldly wise, but he clearly cannot be considered
an innovator. In this respect he differs considerably
from his younger colleague and possible successor, the
brilliant Urso of Calabria, whose name is frequently
linked with that of Maurus. Urso is basically a
theoretician and philosopher who fell completely
under the spell of the new logic; nothing is more revealing than a comparison of Urso's *Compendium
de Urinis* with Maurus's famous work on the same
subject. The *Regulae Urinarum,* as we have seen, is
a straightforward textbook exposition which outlines
and explains the signs to be derived from inspection
of the urine-glass and attempts to correlate these
with a known pathologic process. The style is always
clear and often aphoristic, yet the patient is never
forgotten nor is Maurus too proud to recommend the
diuretics prepared by the herb-gathering *mulieres
Salernitanae.*

Urso's tract seems more concerned with precise
formulation of the material in a logical arrangement
than with any practical application. The subtle
distinctions, excessive refinements, and endless defini-

---

[117] Commentary on the *Isagoge* of Johannitius (B.N. lat.
18499 2rA).
[118] Our text 30.22; *CS* 4: pp. 518, 557.
[119] Riesman, p. 35.

tions reveal a mind obsessed with a desire for ultimate clarity and truth. Yet this tendency toward abstract speculation precludes any serious interest in external nature, and Urso's entire approach seems sterile and impersonal.

We are not yet in a position to assess Maurus's final place in the history of medieval medicine. After all his works have been edited and published, he may well prove to have been one of the most prolific of medieval medical writers. Even a decision as to the originality of his commentaries on Hippocrates must now await a comparison with earlier commentaries on these identical texts. Finally, because both Lawn and Birkenmajer have already stressed the strong Aristotelian element in Maurus's commentary on the *Isagoge* of Johannitius, this work—whose complete publication is particularly to be desired—may easily prove to be his most stimulating contribution to the theory of medicine and to the history of philosophy.

COMMENTARIUS MAURI SALERNITANI IN LIBRUM PROGNOSTICORUM HIPPOCRATICUM LATINUM RECENSUIT BREVIQUE ADNOTATIONE CRITICA INSTRUXIT

Morris Harold Saffron

SIGLA

[Numeri uncis inclusi spectant ad folia columnasque manuscripti latini 18499 Parisini, apud Bibliothecam Nationalem; verba litteraeque uncis quadratis inclusae textus restaurandi causa interposita sunt; textusque Hippocratis in quem exposuit Maurus in litteris italicis est.

Vat = Codex Vaticanus latinus 4477]

1. Pronosticorum Ypocratis fulgor inextricabilis arcam mentis funditus irradians et illustrans humane dispositionis certa metitur indicia secreta, nec rimatur ea longevitate temporis experiendo perscribens. Inquisita namque tripplicitate materie circa quam generalis versatur scientia significatio[1] quo ad quod reliqua videtur precellere, cum corporis habitum triplicem dispositionem et eius causam triplicem, tripliciter reseret et reserando dilucidet. Quod necessarium ducens Ypocrates de significationibus speciale opus ab aliis suis operationibus excerpsum[2] composuit, quod in presentiarum legendum assumpsimus. In cuius compendioso principio ista requiruntur: materia, intentio, intentionis causa, utilitas, suppositio operis, eiusdem particio, ordo tractandi et libri titulus. Huius auctoris materia sunt illa tria, scilicet, corporis forma, actio et superfluitas. Omne namque signum aut sumitur a forma corporis aut ab actionibus eius aut superfluitatibus. Intentio eius est per haec tria certitudinem signorum future mortis vel vite prolixitatis seu brevitatis maxime acutorum et peracutorum morborum evidenter ostendere. Causa intentionis fuit empiricorum et methoycorum temeritas seu repugnantia, qui non attendentes signa neque causas egritudinum de brevi longam faciebant egritudinem de curabili incurabilem, vel eius intentio fuit humani corporis dignitas gratia cuius huius voluminis et aliorum inventa est tractatio. Utilitas eius est preteritarum dispositionum humani corporis rememoratio, presentium demonstratio, futurarum precognitio. Supponitur liber iste practice quia per (123rB) eam signorum habeatur noticia, per practicam medicine, per medicinam phisice, per phisicam theorice, per theoricam[3] spectat [ad] philosophiam. Partitur hoc opus in tres particulas gratia trium virtutum, quarum primam ascribimus virtuti animali, secundam naturali, terciam vero spirituali. Ordo tractandi talis est: auctor premittit prologum in quo medicum logicum ad hanc artem invitat per utile et honestum, per contemplationem universalium et particularium, deinde accedit ad suam intentionem et tractat in prima particula de hiis que sumentur secundum vigorem vel vitium virtutis animalis, in secunda naturalis, in tercia spiritualis. Titulus talis est: Incipit liber pronosticorum. Cum enim communiter in hoc libro de signis tam demonstrativis quam rememorativis quam etiam pronosticis tractet, librum suum potius a pronosticis intitulavit tanquam a dignioribus. Digniora enim sunt pronostica preteritis et demonstrativis nam, ut ait Galenus, demonstrativorum quidem magna est utilitas, rememorativorum vero maior, pronosticorum vero maxima. Et ex hoc patet quod pronostica differre possumus vel omnino evertere, preterita vero si sint vel non sint permutare impossible, vel intitulavit librum suum a pronosticis tanquam a signis, pronosticum nil aliud sonat apud antiquos quam signum. Unde Galenus in *Tegni* vocat omnia signa pronostica tam demonstrativa quam rememorativa.

2. *Omnis et cetera:* Operi suo Ypocrates praetermittit proemium more recte scribentium opus suum extollendo multiplici commendatione, hic autem reddit lectorem docilem benivolum et attentum—docilem dum dicit in singulis egritudinibus preterita, presentia et futura cognoscat; benivolum dum utilitatem insinuat; [et] attentum dum dicit studio artis medicine, ex hoc autem opere, medicus laudem et gloriam et amicorum sibi comparat copiam. Gloriam dum preterita rememorans, presentia demonstrans et futura predicans; laudem dum egrum saluti restituit quem mortis urget metus quem dolor excruciat (123vA) infinitus; amicorum copiam quia unum sanans medetur omnibus quos dolor unius excruciabat. *Omnis qui medicine artis studio seu gloriam seu delectabilem:* studium est vehemens animi applicatio ad aliquid peragendum summa cum voluntate, gloria est frequens fama cum laude, *adeo prudentium regulis minuat suam rationem:*[4] id est philosophorum, *ut in singulis valitudinibus,*[5] id est egritudinibus. Dicitur egritudo valitudo eo quod de egritudine quid valeat natura adversus morbum an

---

[1] *fortasse* significatioque *vice* significatio quo
[2] *fortasse* exerptum *vice* excerpsum
[3] per theoricam philosophie *Vat 37rA*

[4] rationem suam in se rationabilem mutuat *Vat 37rB*
[5] valetudinibus *Vat 37rB*

22

morbus adversus naturam demonstratur, vel dicitur egritudo valitudo ab illo ultimo valde antiquorum, vel dicitur valitudo per contrarium non quod valitudinem conferat sed quia aufert. *Preterita rememorando presentia* demonstrando et *futura pronosticando cognoscat et egro revelet quod de se* [ipso] *minime presenserit:* laudat magis pronostica, magnum est enim preterita rememorare, maius presentia demonstrare, maxime[6] futura predicere. *Si enim per eum cognoverit:* ut predicat ea que debet pati; *certius se illi committit:* confidens in eo tanquam in actore[7] sue salutis, credens ei eger omnia cum aviditate facit sicque fit ut egri confidentia medicine iuvet offitium. *Finisque medicine existit laudabilis:* finis alius medico alius egro pertinet, medico ut conservet, preservet et curet, egro ut curetur et preservetur, hunc ergo finem non semper consequitur medicus.   Unde Boetius: nec medicus semper curabit, sed nec orator semper persuadebit nec sophista semper decipiet, sed si nil ex contingentibus omiserit non minus suum finem consecutum esse censemus. Est et alius finis quem semper debet consequi medicus ut curet curari possibiles et morituros solis signis pronosticis derelinquat. *Cum auc*[tor] *in singulis,* scilicet egritudinibus, *bene perpendit quamvis omnes minime curare possit,* ideo hoc additur ut medicus non credat (123vB) quod hunc finem curandi semper exsequitur sed alium finem. *Quod si omnes posset curare jam non futuri previsor sed divinus diceretur*[8] *no*[bilior], id est, prophetis. *Verum quia vi et acumine et egritudinis*[9] *hunc repente mori contingit:* id est, violento acumine egritudinis.   Duobus enim modis moritur, quis ex egritudine a suo acumine aut sua cruditate vel viscositate, unde dum dixit *vi* notavit viscositatem, dum dixit acumine furiositate[m] medicine[10] ostendit. Mors alias naturalis alias casualis: naturalis que habet prefixum terminum de qua dicitur statuisti terminos eius qui preteriri non poterunt, mors casualis est quam ne eveniat prohibere possumus. *Alium vero medicine prevenit apparatus et vix dieculam vite adicit:* morte, scilicet, casuali. *Interest ergo artificis,* id est, ad utilitatem spectat medicine, *si vires egri atque egritudinis bene perpendit:* debet autem medicus in disgnoscendis: signis semper laborare ut mortem vel vitam vel tarde venturarum[11] per signorum noticiam demonstret. *Est etiam quoddam celeste,* quidam dicunt celeste signum, id est, celatum, quod si sciret medicus mortem vel vitam cito prediceret, vel dicimus quod hic invitat nos auctor ad astronomiam per quam presentia preterita et futura disnoscimus, ideoque est celestium scientia *in quo,* id est, in qua ipsum medicum oportet previdere. *Cuius si tanta fuerit prudentia*[12] *admi*[rabilis] *est nimiumque stu*[penda]: per id enim signum

future mortis vel vite possunt haberi indicia. *Nonne illius est ut futurum periculum vel non omnino prohibeat,* id est, ad illius spectat offitium; *vel competenti adminiculo to*[lerabilus] *fa*[ciat],[13] id est, moderamine. Licet enim eger non possit a morte liberari tamen medicus debet talia sibi dare ut levior videatur; *et si morituro mortem alii vero salutem pronunciet numquid accu*[sationem] *in altero*[14] *promeretur:* non, quia hoc spectat ad suam artem ut morituro mortem, victuro salutem pronunciet.

PARTICULA PRIMA

3. [*Prognostics* I] *Oportet et cetera:* premisso prologo Ypocrates redit ad suam intentionem, est enim eius intentio tractare de signis acutarum egritudinum quod ex tenore littere patet dum dicit: oportet medicum sollicitum fieri circa acutas egritudines.   Hic autem prime particule est principium quam virtuti assignamus animali, non propter quod incohet a cerebro quod est sedes virtutis animalis sed quia hic ponuntur signa que sumuntur secundum vigorem vel vitium virtutis animalis.   Tractat hic de signis acutorum et peracutorum morborum quorum tempora difficilia sunt ad cognoscendum sic[15] eorum tempora cognoscuntur difficile.   Constant[inus] autem in libro febrium VIIII genera ponit signorum laudabilium vel inlaudabilium.   Primum signum laudabile est fortitudo egri morbum suum tollerare potentis, eius contrarium est egri debilitas morbum suum tollerare nequeuntis. Secundum signum laudabile est facilitas motus corporis et quorumlibet membrorum eius etiam tamen cum moderantia, eius contrarium inlaudabile est gravitas tocius corporis et quorumlibet membrorum eius.   Tercium signum laudabile est effigies egri sibi sano similis, eius contrarium est effigies egri sibi sano dissimilis.   Quartum signum laudabile est sanitas mentis et bonus habitus ad oblationes, eius signum contrarium est mentis insania et malus habitus ad oblationes.   Quintum signum laudabile est sompni equalitas.[16]   Sextum signum laudabile est facilitas spiritus, id est, facilis actio inspirandi et exspirandi, eius contrarium est spiritus difficultas.   Iuxta illud spiritus si frequens fuerit ea que circa diafragma sunt egrotare significat.   Septimum signum laudabile est equalitas pulsus, eius contrarium est pulsus inequalitas.   Octavum signum laudabile est fortitudo caloris circa locum excoctionis materiei cum fortitudine virtutis digestive, eius contrarium est debilitas caloris circa locum excoctionis cum debilitate virtutis digestive.   Nonum signum laudabile competens expulsio (124rB) materiei per convenientes regiones, eius contrarium est incompetens expulsio materiei et [per] convenientes regiones.   Quandoquidem medicus

---

[6] *fortasse* maximum *vice* maxime
[7] *fortasse* auctore *vice* actore
[8] sed divinis philosophis *Vat 37rB*
[9] et *ante* egritudinis *fortasse delendum*
[10] materie *vice* medicine *Vat 37B, fortasse recte*
[11] venturam *Vat 37rB*
[12] providentia *Vat 37rB*

[13] tollerabilis fiat *Vat 37rB*
[14] in aliquo *Vat 37rB*
[15] *fortasse* si *vice* sic
[16] enim contrarium est inequalitas sompni *additur post* equalitas *Vat 37rA*

morituro finem victuro salutem pronunciat, et accusationem non promeretur. In altero ne promereatur *oportet esse solli[citum] circa acu[tas] egri[tudines] primo egri faciem perno[tabis]*: ut dictum est superius omnis significatio aut sumitur ex forma corporis aut ex significationibus eius aut ex superfluitatibus. Quia ergo digniora sunt signa, primo agit de signis que sumuntur ex forma corporis nam tria sunt que conferant rei, id esse, quod est: Opifex, substantia et forma. Quorum scilicet opifex primordialis est et dignius ceteris, a quo reliqua duo suam causaliter traxere originem; secundum, scilicet substantia, vicem optinet materie atque subiecti a quo nulla in rebus est differentia, neque numerus neque discretio. Forma vero adveniens substantiis[17] eas ad invicem discrevit easque specificando sub certo rerum genere collocavit. Agens de signis que sumuntur secundum formam corporis primo agit de signis que sumuntur ex forma faciei, vel quia facies primo videntibus occurrit, vel quia habet teneram et delicatam substantiam unde a qualibet qualitate excedente et a quolibet humore inficiente alteratur et inficitur, ut est videri in yctericia quia primo color viridis apparet in facie quam in alia parte corporis, vel est alia causa quia duo sunt potissima que declarant statum et consistentiam hominis, vita, scilicet et sensus, quorum utrumque in facie consideratur: vita scilicet per inspirationem et exspirationem; sensus considerantur in facie quia fere quinque sensus in facie collocantur. *Primo enim egri fac[iem] perno-[tabis]*: hoc modo *utrum sit sano similis*, per quod declarantur quod non plurimum eger sit permutatus a priori consistentia, unde fortitudo egri morbum suum tollerare potentis declaratur. Sed sunt quidam egri similes sanis qui laborant pleuresi vel perypleumonia qui propter suc(124vA)cessionem spiritualium rubent parte egritudinis, ideo dicit *sibi sano similis* ut si fuerit flegmaticus vel melancolicus pallens in sanitate palleat in egritudine, si rubuerit in sanitate proportionaliter in egritudine. *Quod optimum est* quia duo signa laudabilia, per hoc declaratur effigies sibi sano similis, ecce primum signum laudabile; fortitudo infirmi ecce tercium[18] signum laudabile. *Signum est pessimum* si effigies egri sit sano dissimilis et debilitas infirmi morbum suum tolerare non potentis, haec enim duo signa pessima sunt. Et diceret aliquis que sunt particularis[19] malum denotantia que in facie denotantur: *ut si nares acute fuerint;* acuitas narium signum est accidentalis caloris consumentis substantialem humiditatem narium. Nares etiam participant quadam naturali humiditate ipsas relaxante. *Oculi concavi* vel propter exuberantiam accidentalis caloris consumentis et dissolventis humiditatem oculorum vel propter suffocationem spiritualium. In pulmone enim dum consumitur substantialis humiditas nervi contrahuntur, et quia nervi pulmonis habent colligantiam cum oculis

unde dum nervi illi contrahuntur et oculi quare apparent concavi, sicut enim in suspensis oculi foras resiliunt its in suffocatis oculi interius contrahuntur. *Timpora plana*, id est, concava, propter substantialem humiditatem exaustam ex febrili calore. *Aures frigide et contracte:* frigiditas aurium in acuta egritudine aut significat defectum naturalis caloris aut acutum apostema natum [in] intrinsecis aut defectum virtutis nutrientis. Defectum naturalis caloris quia calor illas partes primo derelinquit quas ultimo expeciit sed ultimo expeciit aures, unde cum deficit aures frigescunt ex acuto apostemate nato in intrinsecis. Aures frigescunt quia dum patiuntur interiora membra tamquam nobilia, exteriora minus nobilia mittunt spiritum et calorem ad intrinseca unde extrin(124vB)seca spiritu et calore pauperata frigescunt. Frigiditas aurium declarat defectum virtutis nutrientis nam dum debitum nutrimentum subministratur membris calor non inveniens fomentum deficit, unde aures frigescunt et contracte propter contractionem nervorum, et pulpe earum inverse propter profundam corruptionem caloris augentis in humiditate et consumentis. *Frons arida et tensa:* quia si in membris expositis haec fiunt quid fiet interius maius malum propter maiorem consumptionem. *Tocius co[lor] faciei viridis* propter adustionem; *sive niger*, quod significat vel adustionem vel mortificationem, *sive pallidus*, quod significat principium mortificationis, *sive plumbeus*, quod significat profundam mortificationem. *Que si sic fuerint in principio egritudinis oportet inquiri*, id est, de principio medicine inquirere, quia huius sinthomata predicta aut eveniunt in egritudinibus et non ex egritudinis proprietete, si proveniant in egritudine et ex proprietate egritudinis ut in vigiliis precedentibus non sunt verenda. Ex vigiliis corpus maceratur unde predicta sinthomata possunt emergere et ideo dicit *an vigilie multe precesserint an ven[tris] mul[te] solutiones:* ex solutione ventris possunt predicta emergere sinthomata, *an ieiunii labo[res]*, eodem modo in ieiuniis laborantibus talia sinthomata accidunt. *Et si aliquid cognoveris precessisse aut ven[tris] solutiones et cetera minus periculum vere[beris]:* iam talia signa sunt in egritudine et non ex egritudinis proprietate, vel non indicat nobis precedens nox. *Quod si in precedenti die et nocte quicquam horum substinuerit:* eveniunt sinthomata ex proprietate egritudinis, *non multum periculum sperabis si vero nichil horum cognoveris*, id est, nulla talia sinthomata, non provenientia ex proprietate egritudinis, *mortis signum sperabis* quia proveniunt in egritudine et egritudinis proprietate et sic huius[modi] egritudo triduana fuerint,[20] id est, huius[modi] egra dispositio signorum per tres dies apparuerint[21] quod (125rA) precesserint labores. *Non minus periculum sperabis* quia sunt conversa in habitum, et *omnia que sunt inquirenda circa corpus perquires:* non tamen predicta sunt inquirenda sed que circa corpus et oculos;

[17] subiectis *vice* substantiis *Vat 37vA*
[18] *fortasse* secundum *vice* tercium
[19] *fortasse* particularia *vice* particularis

[20] huiusmodi . . . fuerit *Vat 38rA*
[21] apparuerit *Vat 38rA*

et *enim si lumen effu[gerint]*, quod lumen effugiunt
signum est paucitatis visibilis spiritus, quia ex claritate
extrinseca aëris propter acuitatem et debilitatem disgregatur, unde fertur sensibilis lesio et sic lumen effugiunt, vel dicendum quod obscuritas est visus congregativa et claritas visus disgregativa et omnis res agens
in aliud passionem suscipit a re in qua agit.   Insanis
ergo hominibus tum quia visibilis spiritus est multus et
fortis tum quia instrumenta visus sunt fortissima
quamvis passionem suscipiant.   Tamen si non passionem tolerant egri autem passionem sine magna
molestia nequeunt suscipere, tum quia spiritus visibilis est et paucus unde cito disgregatur, tum quia instrumenta sunt debilia multum ideoque lum[en] effu-
[giunt], nolen[tes] lacri[mas] effu[ndunt] quod
significat fortem actionem circa substantialem humiditatem cerebri que ab eo dissoluta dum mittitur ad
oculos per poros eorum exiens distillat in lacrimas.
Aut foris tanquam in suffocatione[22] *prominueri[n]t*
propter suffocationem in spiritualibus ex [hu]miditate
replente spiritualia.   Spiritus tanquam corpora subtilia cedunt humoribus et cum impetu veniunt ad
oculos cum [quibus] habent colligantiam unde foras
resiliunt.   *Aut alter altero minor appa[ruerit]*: propter
consumptionem substantialis humiditatis alterius et
precipue sinistri, quia si calor accidentalis tanti pre-
valuerit in sinistra parte, frigiditas multo plus pre-
valuerit[23] in dextra, et *al[ba] eorum in sanguinea com-
[mutata] fuerint*, quod signum est acute materiei a qua
actua resolvitur fumositas que veniens ad oculos
abrumpit venas oculorum et sic sanguis exit unde
rubor adest oculorum; vel quia ex suffocatione spiritualium spiritus cum sanguine mittuntur ad oculos et
eius suppositione alba eorum videtur sanguinea.   *Aut
tanquam ve[ne] nigrio[ris]* que declarant mor (125rB)-
tificationem vel adustionem, *aut palloris* que declarant
principium mortificationis.   *Intus viso fuerint et lipi-
tudinem habundaverit*:[24] hoc significat fortem calorem
profunditus agentem in cerebrum et dissolventem
ipsum, substantialis humiditas veniens ad oculos et ab
exteriori aëre desiccatur et efficitur lippitudo.   Et
instabi[les] fuerint: instabilitas oculorum triplici ex
causa habet fieri, vel propter debilitatem et paucitatem
visibilis spiritus unde disgregatur et sequitur instabilitas, vel quia ab acuta materia acuta resolvitur
fumositas que veniens ad oculos pungit et mordicat
teneram substantiam oculorum, unde ipsi refugiunt
contraria et sic efficiuntur instabiles; vel ex siccitate
sequitur mentis alienatio unde futura est frenesis, unde
fit amentia, et sic movent oculos huc illuc.   *Et tremuli,*
quia significat debilitatem virtutis regitive oculorum
unde tremuli, sicut est videri in paraliticis.   *Aut extra
nimis extiterint*, hoc ideo dicit ut aliud addat *aut intus
mul[tum] delituerint*, hoc significat fortem calorem
consumentem substantialem humiditatem oculorum

qua consumpta ipsi minorantur quare videntur delites-
cere; vel significat substantialem nervorum humiditatem opticorum forti calore consumptam, unde nervi
ipsi contrahuntur; contractis, contrahuntur oculi quibus sunt alligati et hoc significat futurum spasmum
ex inanitione.   Et *tota fa[cies] ori[bilis] appa[ruerit]
livida*, vel viridis quod significat tocius nature habitu-
dinis immutationes.   *Hec omnia peri[culosa] et mor-
[talia] iudi[cabis.]   Oportet videri quid de oculis in
sompnis vide[atur]*: auctor in precedentibus sufficienter pronosticatus est circa dispositionem oculorum in
vigiliis, nunc intendit pronosticari circa dispositionem
eorumdem in sompno, quia ex dispositione eorum in
sompno future mortis vel vite eliciuntur pronostica.
Palpebre sunt membra cartillaginosa oculos coöperi-
entia ipsos ab exteriori nocumento defendentia.   Hec
igitur membra, scilicet palpebre, colligantiam habent
cum duobus (125vA) panniculis cerebrum ab exteriori
nocumento defendentibus, scilicet cum dura matre et
pia matre, unde cum liquorosa fumositas a cibis et
potibus resolvitur et petens cerebrum, tanquam tocius
corporis caminum, predictos panniculos humectat et
remollit et homo vigiliis privatur; per humectationem
et relaxationem ipsorum panniculorum habentium
colligantiam cum palpebris palpebrarum fit humecta-
tio, relaxatio et aggravatio et oculos coöperiunt.   Sed
contingit quandoque quod quidam habent magnos oculos et palpebras curtas, quidam ex solutione ventris
habent curtas palpebras.   Sed neque ex consuetudine
habent curtas palpebras ut in habentibus oculos magnos et apparet al[ba] oculorum, vel ex fluxu ventris
contingit palpebrarum curvitas, mortalia sunt talia
signa; significatur enim quod substantialis humiditas
resoluta a cibis et potibus que debebat humectare panniculos, scilicet duram matrem et piam matrem, et
propter collimitantiam panniculorum ad palpebras
palpebras debebant humectare et extendere, quod fit
exausta actione febrilis caloris substantialis humiditas
nervorum venientium ad palpebras, unde dum contrahuntur nervi et palpebre contrahuntur quibus sunt
alligati, et sic palpebre sunt semicluse, et si membra
exposita sunt consumpta quid iam calor fecit in intrinsecis combuxit intrinseca, et hoc est quod dixit auctor.
Si enim sola al[ba] vi[deantur] subclu[sis] pal[pebris]
quare pocius alba videatur quam nigra dicimus quoniam dum palpebre semicluduntur oculum non claudunt
alba sed nigra similiter alba apparent.   *Neque solutio
aut per se*, id est, non eveniat per solutionem sponta-
neam; *sive per catarticum precessit*, id est, non eveniat
ex artificiali; *neque ex consuetudine hoc evenit*, ut in
habentibus oculos magnos et palpebras curtas, *mor[tis]
significa[tiones] ti[mebis]*; quia si hoc fit in viridi quid
fiet (125vB) in arido, vel fecit[25] combuxit, et *si palpe-
[bre] inverse fuerint* ex consumptione substantialis
humiditatis ipsarum unde inverse appa[rent] *aut
livide* ex mortificatione; *sive labra similiter fu[erint]
livi[da]*, propter mortificationem, *aut nares distor[te]*,

---

[22] Aut fortis tanquam in suffocato *Vat 38rA*
[23] tantum prevaluit *Vat 38rA*
[24] habuerint *Vat 38rA*

[25] *fortasse* vel facto: *MS habet* f̄ct

propter contractionem nervorum nares distorquentur, *hiis signiis sive solis,* id est, per se apparentibus *sive cum predictis* superius enumeratis *mortem proximam iudicabis.*

4. [*Prognostics* III] *Bonum est egrum et cetera:* circa scema iacendi auctor pronosticatur quia ex dispositione iacendi future mortis vel vite elitiuntur pronostica. Dicit auctor: *bonum est egrum inve[nire] iacen-[tem] aut in dextro aut in sinistro latere.* Per hoc quod aliquis libere et sine molestia iacet super utrumque latus removetur a nobis suspectio apostematum in ambobus lateribus minime contingentium vel in altero illorum laterum unde pro abscentia apostematum removetur suffocationis et succensionis spiritualium suspectio, dum non fit suffocatio homo libere potest sedere super utrumque latus, dum non fit succensio spiritualium homo libere potest attrahere aërem ad mitigationem innati caloris et sic secure potest sedere super utrumque latus. Sed cum sit bonum sedere supra utrumque latus an sit melius in dextro an in sinistro. Dicimus hec previsa ratione in dextra parte est epar et idem facit epar suppositum stomacho quod ignis lebeti ex vicinia epatis ad stomachum et bona fit digestio in stomacho et competens in epate unde congrua humiditas fit generatio decens et oportuna spirituum reparatio unde virtu[tes] melius peragunt suas actiones. Vel est alia causa quare melius sit iacere in dextro latere quam in sinistro, quia reumatica causa magis consuevit moveri in sompno quam in vigiliis. In sompno enim ex reumatica causa naturalis ad intrinseca ca[loris] fit confortatio eiusdem[que] multiplicatio; unde calore multiplicato humores dissolvuntur. Ex dis(126rA)solutione eorum ad spiritualia venientes ad pulmonem, cum sit membrum concavum cavernosum, humiditas effluens in concavitate pulmonis potest retineri sine lesione, quare cum pulmo sit in dextro latere, melius est iacere in dextro latere. Cor positum in sinistro latere non habet nisi parvam concavitatem ut possit effluentem humiditatem substinere sine lesione. *Et manus et pe[des] et cervicem non ut [in] spasmo distenta et contracta:* per hoc quod pedes [et] manus fluxiles[26] sunt fortitudo egri morbum suum tolerare potentis declaratur et *mi[nime] rigid[da],* id est, dura, dum dicit, *et totum corpus in sua positione fluxibile[27]* facilitas motus tocius corporis insinuatur. *Hec habitudo,* id est, constantia, *sanis est fa[miliaris],* quia ita se debent habere sani, et *iacere in modum sani melius est,* sicut consuevit quando sanus erat, ut in sinistro latere in sinistro, si in dextro in dextro, si supinus, supinus, *quia non est signum laudabile egrum in corpore supino iacere,* its tamen si non sit ex consuetudine, vel per hoc declaratur quod adsit collectio in ambobus lateribus quare cum non possit iacere in utroque vel in altero iacet supinus, vel declaratur si subita suffocatio vel succensio spiritualium quare hoc supinus querit aërem frigidum. *Bracchiis et pe[dibus]*

rigi[dis], id est, non equaliter calentibus; et *si re-[pente] se a ca[pite] lec[ti] ad pe[des] iacta[verit]:* ex hoc declaratur amentia ex humore collecto ad frenesim. Dum homo desipit huc atque illuc flectitur, vel quia sequitur succensio spiritualium unde querit liberum aërem et ideo movetur a capite lecti ad pedes. *Malum non dubitabilis[28]* vel propter predicta vel propter amentiam. *Et si pe[des] nu[dos]* vel a carne vel a pannis, quia si consumpsit ca[lorem] substantialem humiditatem expositorum membrorum multo magis proximorum, *et tepidos inve[neris],* id est, non equaliter calentes, *et inordi[nate] cum la[bore] cer[vicem],* propter defectum virtu[tis] regitive, *atque pedes iacta-[verit] pessi[mum] est* et (126rB) *angustie signum,* quia debilitas infirmi morbum suum tolerare nequeuntis perpenditur.

5. *Eger si iacuerit reiecta cer[vice]:* ponit ad huc auctor signa que sumuntur ex forma corporis mortem proximam minantia dicens, *eger si iacuerit reiecta cer-[vice]* ex debilitate virtu[tis] ipsius capitis unde egro capud ad molem est et sarcinam. Et *ore aperto,* hoc contingit vel ex consumptione nervorum venientium ad inferiorem molem vel contingit ex suffocatione spiritualium unde aperit ut attrahat frigidum aërem ex suffocatione ad vitandam suffocationem os aperit. *Pedibus tortis:* propter contractionem nervorum venientium ad pedes ex humiditate consumpta in nervis contrahuntur nervi et pedes distorquentur. *Aut si sup[ra] ven[trem] preter solitum iacuerit:* preter consuetudinem in hoc quod iacet supra ventrem, vel supra proter amentiam quia nescit quid faciat, vel propter presentiam acuti apostematis nati in ventre. Dum enim acuta materia collecta ad apostema inducit dolorem patiens comprimit ventrem ut stupor inducatur et insensibilitas et sic dolor non sentitur et inde dicit causam unde proveniat. *Malum enim est et alie[nationem] sive do[lorem] significat,* propter acutum apostema natum interius. *Et si in angusto[29] egritudinis re[pente] ste[terit]),* cum quadam mentis insania. *In omni acuta egritudine malum* est sanire quia raptum significat materiei ad superiora. *In peripleumonia pessimum,* quia pulmo ubi contingit peripleumonia liberos habet meatus ad cerebrum unde de facili materia levigatur et petit cerebrum et colligitur ad apostema freneticum.

6. *Frendere dentibus in fe[bribus] et cetera:* auctor intendit pronosticari circa frendorum dentium, frendor dentium est ipsorum motus ex alterutra collisione eorumdem proveniens, sed frendor dentium alius voluntarius, alius involuntarius. Voluntarius qui fit ab egro vel ut astantes terreat vel ut eos (126vA) moveat ad risum vel contingit ex acuta materia actione caloris in fumum dissoluta, et fumus tanquam res subtilis mittitur ad gingivas, unde pungendo et mordicando gingivas inducit dolorem in gingivis; ad vitandum illum dolorem movet quis dentes et dentibus stridet ut in-

---

[26] *fortasse* flexiles *vice* fluxiles
[27] flexibile *vice* fluxibile *Vat 38rB*

[28] *fortasse* dubitabile *vice* dubitabilis
[29] augmento *Vat 38vA*

nascatur stupor et [in]sensibilitas. Involuntarius habet fieri ex consumptione nervorum venientium ad inferiorem molam unde dum nervi contrahuntur inferior mola contrahitur et sic superior ex alterutra collisione inferioris mole ad superiorem. Homo stridet dentibus, talis stridor dentium malus est quia significat insaniam et raptus materiei ad superiora. Dicit ergo, *fren[dere] den[tibus] in fe[bribus] preter solitum*, id est, preter consuetudinem, sicut quidam qui habent ventrem parvum et stomachum indiscrete sumunt cibaria dum fit fluctuatio in stomacho quia cibaria non possunt retineri, nervi venientes ad inferiorem molam replentur et sic stridor dentium. *Nec a puero*, id est, in puero febricitanti: in puero febricitanti non est verendum si adsit stridor dentium, quia ipsi[30] plurima humiditate et actione caloris participat unde dum dissolvitur humiditas replentur nervi qui veniunt ad molam inferiorem et sic stridor dentium. *Mortem vel maniam significat*, et si non sit ex consuetudine vel in puero.

7. *Si in egro cor[pore] fiat an[trax]*: circa mortifera apostema provenientia in febribus acutis ex materia super accensa intendit auctor pronosticari. Natura ex febribus acutis debilitata non potest perfecte crisim operari. Facit ergo quod potest, materiam nocivam a nobilibus membris ad ignobilia transmittit et ibi obvolvitur crustula et ad apostema colligitur. Tale apostema vel tale evenientia[31] in febribus acutis aut habet fieri ex colera aut ex sanguine. Factum ex colera dicitur antrax vel ab antro quia locus quem possidet est in modum antri vel antrax dicitur quia antrum protendit[32] co[lor]. Factum ex sangui[ne] dicitur carbunculus in modum car(126vB)bonis accensi quia rubrum portendit co[lorem]. Apostema factum ex colera nigrum portendit co[lorem] quia siccitas exacuendo calorem ut sit eius sima caloris,[33] ignitus agit ad denigrationem ut est videri in carbone denigrato. Factum ex sanguine portendit rubrum co[lorem] quia humiditas sanguinis contradicendo[34] siccitati, siccitas non potest co[lorem] exacuere unde rubeus co[lor]. Sed ut aliquis sciat utrum fiat vi nature vel vi sinthomatis attendendum est quia si locum quem possidet non derelinquat nisi cum eiectione nocive materiei ad exteriora fiunt vi nature, si delitescat attendendum est etiam vel locum quem derelinquat si apparuerit ibi co[lor] factus ex discursu hu[moris] bonum est et fit vi nature quia calor naturalis confortatus consumpsit totam nocivam materiam unde co[lor] nocivi humoris non debet apparere. Sed si signum vestigii ibi apparuerit fit ibi vi sinthomatis, sed dimisit ibi materia suos satellites et ipsa materia levigata et transit ad aliquod membrum principale [et] mortem inducit, et hoc est quod dicit. *Si in egro corpore fit*

antrax, quia in neutro non est verendum, *vel carbunculus precesse[rit] sive egritudini supervenit*, quia aliquando supervenit aliquando non *opus attendere est* utrum superveniat vel non. *Quod si exsiccatus fuerit*, hoc est delitescat, et *co[lorem] vi[ridem]* propter adustionem signum est quod fit vi sinthomatis; *vel ci-[trinum] co[lorem]*, signum quod fiat ex colera, *vel levi[dum]*[35] propter mortificationem; *co[lorem] pretulerit mor[tem] proximam dicit* propter raptum materiei ad cerebrum nobile et eius dissipando substantiam mortem inducit.

8. [*Prognostics IV*] *Manuum mo[bilitatis] signa sic praeno[tabis]*: circa mobilitatem manuum in acuta febre et apostemate peripleumoniaco auctor pronosticari intendit, quia ex motione manuum future mortis vel vite eliciuntur pronostica. *In fe[bre] acuta in peripleumonia*: in febre acuta materia rapitur ad superiora ex caloris[36] dissolventis materiam, unde materia rapitur ad superiora sed hoc modo manum suam commoverit aliquis tanquam aliquid collecturus. No[tatur] est signum acute materiei pungentis (127rA) et mordicantis teneram et nobilem substantiam faciei unde pro punctura et mordicatione manum ad faciem inicit aliquid collecturus. Similiter peripleumonia, quia pulmo liberos habet meatus ad superiora unde dum materia transit pro violentia materiei manum ponit ad faciem. *In fre[nesi] non vera*: non vera frenesis hic dicitur facta ex humoribus spiritum visibilem inficientibus, et *in do[lore] ca[pitis] si ma[nus] ad fa[ciem] tu[lerit]* propter raptum materiei ad superiora. *Tam quidlibet tanquam positu[rus]* propter mordicationem et puncturam vitandam ponit manum ad faciem ac si aliquid posuisset, *vel quasi aliquid col-[lecturus] [h]ac et illac quesierit*: per hoc significatur dispersio materiei, *vel de vestibus aliquid evulserit*, propter fumositates subtiles inficientes spiritum visibilem represententantes musculas vel ceu festucas. *De paritiis decersepserit*[37] *pess[imum] et mor[tale] est* talia enim signa minantia sunt futuram frenesim.

9. [*Prognostics V*] *Spiritus si fre[quens] sit et cetera*: circa actionem inspirandi intentio actoris est pronosticari, dicens, *spiritus si fre[quens]*, spiritus multipliciter accipitur pro actione inspirandi et respirandi, accipitur pro aëre inspirato et respirato ut cum dicitur sudem per os et na[res] frigidum exierit. Accipitur pro quadam subtili et aërea substantia virtu[tes] corporis excitante et cetera: hic ut dictum est accipitur pro actione inspirandi et respirandi. Sed actio inspirandi et respirandi aut est magna aut parva aut frequens aut rara. Multa fit per calorem, parva fit per frigiditatem, rara per humiditatem, frequens per siccitatem. Magna fit per caliditatem hoc modo, nam dum spiritualia distemperantur in multo ca[lore] cor pro multa distemperantia caloris querit attrahere multum de aëre frigido, sed multus aër non potest at-

---

[30] *fortasse* ipse *vice* ipsi
[31] *fortasse* eveniens *vice* evenientia
[32] *fortasse* portendit *vice* protendit
[33] *fortasse* carbonis *vice* caloris
[34] *fortasse* contradicens *vice* contradicendo

[35] *fortasse* lividum *vice* levidum
[36] *fortasse* ex [causa] caloris *sive* vi *vice* ex
[37] *fortasse* de parietiis decerpserit

trahi nisi multum dilatetur cor et multa dilatatio multam facit inspirationem et quia multa est dilatatio multa est constrictio et multa constrictio facit magnam respirationem. Vel aliter, calor operatur ad generationem fumositatum (127rB) unde per calorem multe fumositates resolute habente[38] motum ad centrum operantur ad multam dilatationem et multe fumositates parate erant ca[lorem] cordis extinguere. Multa sequitur constrictio ad emissionem fumositatum superfluitatum. Per frigiditatem pauca fit inspiratio et respiratio, nam dum spiritualia distemperantur frigiditas non permittit fieri fumositatum generationem quare multus aër attrahitur ad mitigationem caloris cordis, sed paucus aër facit paucam dilatationem et si pauca est dilatatio pauca inspiratio et quia pauca est dilatatio pauca erit constrictio et sic parva respiratio. Vel quia frigiditas mo[tum] habet ad centrum semper operatur ad parvam inspirationem et respirationem. Frequens fit per siccitatem; siccitas est luna[39] caloris unde exacuendo ca[lore] calor multus operatur ad multam dilatationem sicque siccitas motum habet ad centrum operans ad constrictionem non permittit fieri multam dilatationem unde quod deest ei in quantitate suppletur in temporis vicissitudine. Rara fit per humiditatem: humiditas obtundendo ca[lore] cordis operatur ad raritatem. Dicit ergo, *spiritus si fre[quens] sit*, id est, actio inspirandi et respirandi et *dolor significat*, id est, materia doloris et *succensionem*, unde succenduntur spiritualia *ex dolore*. Fit frequens inspiratio et respiratio nam omnis do[lor] exacuit reuma et ad locum dolentem defluunt humores unde ex multitudine humorum fit coangustatio meatuum ex eo ipso et discursu humorum et spirituum cor frequenter movetur unde frequens inspiratio et respiratio. *In hiis que sunt super diafragma:* antiqui physici interiora humani corporis perscrutantes a diafragmate superius spiritualia, [inferius nutritiva]. Diafragma est quidam panniculus dividens spiritualia a nutritivis. *Quod si sit magnus*, id est, magna inspiratio et respiratio et *cum intermissione*, id est, cum suspirio; est autem suspirium vehemens exspiratio (127vA) cum vehementi exspiratione cum animal debite actionis oblliviscitur. *Aliena[tio] spiritus:* multitudo inspirationis cum intermissione alienationem significat multitudo inspirationis multitudinem cause significat. Intermissio significat ascensum materiei ad superiora unde alienatio, et *sudorem per os et na[res] fri[gidum] exi[erit] mor[tale]*, faciendo simplicem relaxationem et non discretam per spiritum, non intelligamus actionem inspirandi et re[spirandi] sed aërem inspi[ratum] *et re[spiratum frigidum]*; *mor[tale] est* quia significat extinctionem naturalis caloris in corde, unde mors. Mors nichil aliud est quam extinctio naturalis caloris in corde. *Spiritus bonus*, id est, actio inspi[randi] et re[spirandi] et *suo proprio or[dine] cogn[oscitur]*, id est, neque addit

frequentie neque addit magnitudini et habet evidentem sa[lutis] osten[sionem]. *In acuta egritudine que cum febre est*, quia si bona est actio inspirandi et respirandi bona est dispositio cordis quod est necessarium ad vitam et si bona est disposition cordis bona est dispositio membrorum adiacentium.

10. [*Prognostics* VI] *Sudor bo[nus] et lau[dabilis] et cetera:* diximus superius quod omnis significatio aut sumitur ex forma corporis aut ex superfluitatibus aut ex actionibus. Sufficienter egit auctor superius de signis que sumuntur ex forma corporis. Nunc intendit agere de signis que sumuntur ex superfluitatibus. Notandum quod quattuor sunt a corpore exeuntia quorum quodlibet egritudinum membrorum a quibus educitur est significativum: scilicet sputum, egestio, urina et sudor. Sputum est significativum animatorum membrorum spiritualium et stomachi, quando quidem egestio [est] declarativa passionum nutritivorum ut stomachi et intestinorum; urina est declarativa epatis et viarum urinalium; sudor per coniecturam significat dispositionem tocius corporis. Sudor est vapor humidus a corpore dissolutus per poros corporis exiens et cutim[40] humectans. Sudor multipliciter attenditur in quantitate, qualitate, tenuitate et spissitudine in tempore et in loco. In (127vB) quantitate quia aut est multus aut paucus et tam multus quam paucus aut fit vi nature aut fit vi sinthomatis. Multus sudor fit vi nature quando natura materiam bene digestam et divisam a corpore evacuit[41] et per convenientes regiones. Ita tamen quod ex tali eductione eger levior et suavior efficitur, immo in salutem restituitur. Multus vi sinthomatis habet fieri ex multitudine materiei propter membrorum incontinentiam dum membra nequeunt sustinere hu[mores]; pro multitudine, non solum superfluorum humorum fit eductio, immo et bonorum. Paucus vi nature habet fieri quando natura per aliam regionem quam per sudorem evacuavit nocivam materiam, parum remansit in mediis regionibus a qua paucus sudor. Paucus vi sinthomatis habet fieri pro defectu virtu[tis] expulsive. In qualitate consideratur multipliciter, in colore, odore et sapore: si fuerit albi coloris declarat flegmatis naturalis habundantiam, si rubri habundantiam sanguinis, si crocei colere, si lividi melancolie. In odore consideratur: fetidus declarat corruptionem humorum, gravis membrorum. In sapore consideratur nam si fuerit insi[pidi] saporis declarat habundantiam flegmatis naturalis; si dulcis saporis vel habundantiam sanguinis vel flegmatis dulcis; si acetosi vel melancolie vel flegmatis acetosi; si amari habundantiam colere. In tenuitate consideratur nam si fuerit fluidus subtilium et tenuium humorum declarat habundantiam; si fuerit compactus et solidus solidorum et crassorum humorum declarat habundantiam. In qualitate etiam consideratur aliter in caliditate et frigitate nam calidus minorem significat egritudinem frigidus

---

[38] *fortasse* habent *vice* habente
[39] *fortasse* lima *vice* luna

[40] *fortasse* cutem *vice* cutim
[41] *fortasse* evacuat *vice* evacuit

maiorem. In tempore consideratur quia debet fieri in die cretico deputato operi nature, ita tamen quod ex tali eductione eger levior et suavior efficiatur. Consideratur in loco quia debet fieri per totum corpus qui declarat omnimodam eductionem nocivi humoris. Nam si non (128rA) fiat per totum sed in parte corporis ubi sudor ibi narrat egritudinem et frigidus in collo et cervice factus malus est quia significat extinctionem naturalis caloris. *Sudor bo-[nus] et lau[dabilis] qui fit in die cretico in acuta omni egri[tudine]*: qui fit in die deputato operi nature et *egrum liberat*, propter omnimodam eductionem nocivi humoris. *Et est etiam bonus qui fit in toto corpore:* ex hoc declaratur fortitudo virtu[tis] expulsive et *ex eo eger le[vior] et su[avior] effici[tur]*: propter humorem aggravantem naturam corporis debilitatur, ea enim eductione natura corporis suavior et levior efficitur. *Qui vero nil horum fece[rit] hiis corporibus est inutilis:* quia non fit in die cretico egrum non liberat; non fit in toto corpore et ex eo eger non levior non suavior efficitur, immo magis aggravatur pro humore qui retinetur et corpus debilitatur. *Frigidus autem malus:* aut declarat extinctionem caloris naturalis aut habet fieri ex frigida materia que longum tempus expostulat ad sui digestionem, unde ante quam possit digeri ante debilitatur patiens et sic morbus fortius insurgit contra naturam. *Peior si in cervice et capite solo*, frigiditas emergat quia extinctionem naturalis caloris et in capite et per collum in corde: dixit pocius in hiis membris quia ibi viget virtus attractiva utcumque dissolvit hu[mores] unde transeunt in sudorem et sic quidem in acuta febre mortem significat quia extinctionem naturalis caloris. *Cum longa prolixitate:* egri materiam multam, bonum est ergo. [*Prognostics VII*] *Si fuerit in ypo[condriis] sine do[lore]:* circa habitum ypocondriorum auctor intendit pronosticari: ypocondria sunt loca concava, vacuitatem in se habentia sub teneritatibus costarum. Sciendum est quod quadruplicia sunt ypocondria: duo superiora a diafragmate superius et duo inferiora a diafragmate inferius. Superiora ypocondria in dextra parte posita plurima participant concavitate unde ex maiori sui parte continent pulmonem. Superiora in sinistra parte locata non tanta participant (128rB) concavitate continent enim epar.[42] Inferiora ypocondria in sinistra parte posita multa participant concavitate et continent splenem.[43] Contingit quandoque quod humor preter naturam continetur in ypocondriis unde suscipit ebullitionem caloris et obvolvitur crustula et sic fit apostema. Bo[num] est ergo si fuerit in ypocondriis sine dolore; ubi non est dolor, non est discursus humorum, quia sicut ex discursu humorum fit apostema sic et abscentia denegat ne apostematis materia colligatur ad apostema. In eo enim quod sunt ypocondria sine dolore non enim prevalet in ypocon-

driis humor flegmaticus ut fiat dolor extensivus, non colericus ut fiat [dolor] pungitivus et sic decet; *si mollia*, per quod declaratur quod non prevalet siccitas que consumat humiditatem unde mollitie quadam naturali et ypocondria disponuntur; *si bene composite hinc inde bo[na] erunt*, id est, tam inferiores quam superiores, *si bene co[mposite]*, id est, habeant formam propriam quam debet habere *bonum est*, quia non sunt perturbate ab aliquo humore neque aliquis humor ibi descendit ut colligeretur ad apostema. *Si vero fer-[ventes] aut do[lentes]*: propter descensum humoris sanguinei collecti ad apostema; *aut quodam[modo]*[44] *spasmo disten[te]*: propter flegmaticam materiam replentem et extendentem et *inter [se] dissi[miles]*, vel in una flegmatica et in altera melancolica vel in una sit collecta materia in altera non; *in hiis consi[derandum] est* utrum materia collecta ad apostema sit colerica vel sanguinea. *Si enim in aliqua earum pulsus fuerit*, id est saltus, signum est quod materia sit colerica que actione caloris dissolvitur, dissoluta querit exitum, non potest [exire] propter crustulam unde removet crustulam et sic fit pulsus, *angustiam sive ali[enationem] significat:* angustiam materiam significat sanguineam, id est suffocationem, alienationem melancolica, quia materia colerica subtilis est [et] habilis ad dissolutionem, petit superiora et maniam inducit, et *tum in hac egritudine*, id est, in hac collectione unde egritudo provenit. (128vA)

11. *Oculi sunt intuendi:* quia materia inde transit, *quia si mo[biles] ma[niam] appa[ruerint]*:[45] propter puncturam et mordicationem, unde dum puncture contrarium vitare agiliter moventur, *maniam significat* propter raptum materiei ad superiora et inficiendo anteriorem cellulam capitis. *Acu[ta] existente egritudine collectio si affu[erit]*: ut pote si laboraverit febris *in ypo[condriis] cum tu[more] et do[lore] ut ambas ypo-[condria] te[nsa] malum est:* quia unum apostema in uno sufficit ad pernitiem. *Si vero altera earum, que in sinistra est, melior est*, id est, minus mala, non in sinistro ypocondrio superiori sed inferiori sinistro ubi splen consistit quod est membrum ignobile; si esset in sinistro superiori pessimum esset quia ibi est cor quod est membrum ad vitam destinatum. *Que collectio si in principio su[bitam] mor[tem] non intulerit [et si] usque ad XX diem permanserit neque fe[bris] defe-[cerit] nec do[lor]*: propter continuam transmissionem in partem illam *in post*[46] *convertetur*, diuturna actione calor ebulliens materia verteretur in saniem. *Solet huic ac[ute] egri[tudini] infra VII dies uti[liter] flu[xus] san[guinis] e na[ribus] super[venire]:* de summo vigore nature declaratur invenientis novos meatus, inter ceteras determinationes nulla melior ista. *Perquirendum est autem an do[lor] adsit fronti:* ecce dum materia apostematis debet educi, adest dolor frontis propter materiam ascendentem ad superiora:

---

[42] *certissime* cor *vice* epar
[43] In dextro inferiori continetur epar ex maiori parte *post* splenem *additur Vat 39vA.*

[44] quodammodo *Vat 39vB*
[45] si velociter mobiles apparuerint maniam significat *Vat 39vB*
[46] *fortasse* pus *vice* post.

signa sunt pronostica. *Similiter sco[tomia] si affu-*
[erit] quia materia ascendit superius *san[guinis] flu-*
[xum] e na[ribus] enuntiabis: dum fit abruptio venu-
larum et illis potissime *quibus etas est XXXV annorum*
in quibus humor[es] colerici prehabundant.

12. *Apostemate vero molli exis[tente] et cetera:* secundum diversitates humorum collectorum ad apostema intendit auctor pronosticari secundum manierem
varia[m] apostematis, secundum tempus collectionis
et secundum locum apostematum. Aliud sanguineum, aliud colericum, aliud flegmaticum, aliud melancolicum; et prius de sanguineo intendit auctor
ponere et circa ipsum pronosticari, sed contrarius videtur (128vB) Ioannitius quia asserit apostema sanguineum durum et iste dicit esse molle et sub tactu
mutabile, dicit quod sanguis aut naturalis aut innaturalis: naturalis aut in venis aut in artariis. Sanguis
qui est in venis soliditate participat unde apostema
factum ex eo solidum est de quo Ioannitius dicit facto,
scilicet ex tali humore. Ypocrates ponit in hoc loco
de apostemate facto ex sanguine innaturali, de yquore,
unde dicit, *apostemate vero mol[li] exis[tente]* propter
aquosam materiam cuius aquositate relaxatur apostematis essentia et relaxatum mollificatur, et *sine*
do[lore], vel sine doloris vehementia propter materiam
frigidam, unde frigiditate sua pars quam possidet
sensibilitati contradicit, quare talis dolor dicitur sine
dolore, vel quia non habet qualitates dissolutorias et
pernicatorias.[47] Et *sub tactu mu[tabile]*: non quod
tangatur sed si posset tangi tactui cederit pro labili-
tate unde signum foraminis faceret propter essentiam
materiei multam relaxatam per humiditatem. *Con-*
tingit egritudinem terminari in predictis tamen sepius,
id est, per predictam aut per fluxum sanguinis e naribus aut per saniem, *vel in predictis,* in iuvenibus de
quibus fecerat mentionem. *Quod si usque in diem*
LX[48] sic permanserit: in hoc loco intendit pronosticari de apostemate melancolico cuius ruptura propter
sui soliditatem et compactionem differtur ad XL diem.
Quod si *in die XL sic permanserit,* istud non referatur
ad antecedens[49] ad apostema sed ad apostema melancolicum, ut sit simplex relatio et non personalis, *fe-*
[bre] non defi[ciente]: propter perseverantiam apostematis febris commutatur, tale apostema, *in pus con-*
vertetur; ebulliens materia per calorem diuturna actione ipsius vertitur in saniem. *Et omne apostema*
circa ven[trem] ad hunc modum diudicabitur, id est, aut
fiet determinatio ipsius per saniem aut per fluxum sanguinis. *Apostema vero solidum:* hic intendit pronosticari circa apostema colericum quod vocat solidum,
materia enim que colligitur ad tale aspostema calida
est et sicca. Caliditas licet operatur ad dissolutionem,
siccitas operatur ad consum (129rA)ptionem unde operatur ad soliditatem. *Cum do[lore],* id est, doloris
vehementia propter qualitates dissolutorias et pernec-

atorias; *horrendum,* id est, suspitiosum quia insinuat
materiam acutissimam et violentissimam; et *cito mor-*
ti[ferum], solo enim acumine interficit dum aliquod
membrum principale dissipat, vel *horrendum,* id est,
horribili timore timendum vel suspicioso.[50] Quod
autem molle, pronosticatus est auctor circa apostema
sanguineum et colericum nunc intendit pronosticari
circa apostema flegmaticum. Ista que diximus sunt
signa apostematis sanguinei et colerici sed *quod est*
molle et sine do[lore], ut pote flegmaticum, idem videtur dicere quod dixit de apostemate sanguineo, apostemate vero molli existente et sub tactu mutabili et
dicit de flegmatico quod fit *sub tac[tu] cursile,* notandum quod aliud est sub tactu mu[tabile] aliud sub
tactu cursile. Nam sub tactu cursile plus portat
ultimam et summam motionem sub tactu mutabili[51]
et licet notet motionem non tantum *quod autem molle:*
propter humiditatem materiei emollientem. *Sine*
do[lore]: propter frigiditatem prestantem insensibili-
tatem, unde dolor non sentitur, *tardius solvitur quam*
colericum vel tardius mortem inducit. *Apostema vero*
circa ven[trem]: pronosticatur auctor circa quantitatem collectionis secundum varietatem locorum. Ex
varietate locorum ipsum quandoque magis quandoque
minus colligitur; dicit ergo, *apostema vero circa [ven-*
trem] mi[nus] hu[morem] colligit: quia venter non
tanta participat vacuitate vel ibi sunt meatus proclivi
quam quod in ipo[chondriis] quia maiori participant
concavitate et meatus non sunt proclivi, unde in ypocondriis magis colligitur de materia. *Mi[nime]*
omnium quod sub umbili[co]; quia maiori participant
concavitate umbilicus et meatus proclivi. *El[egan-*
tius] est omnibus signum, si sanguinis est effusio quia
et fortitudo nature insinuatur invenientis novos
meatus ad materiei eductionem.[52] *Ex hiis que sunt in*
prenotatis locis: hoc est, sanies que inest predictis locis,
quasi diceret quia melior est (129rB) determinatio
sanguinis quam facta per saniem, quia dum fit sanies
inpossibile est quod non corrumpatur membrum quod
possidet.

13. *Omne apostema diuturnum:* nunc pronosticatur
circa apostema melancolicum ut aliud addat quod dicitur diuturnum quadam prcrogativa ct cxccllcntia,
vel quia fit ex materia frigida et sicca que solida est et
compacta, vel quia habet determinari diuturniori
tempore quam aliud apostema ut pote in XL[53] die.
Omne apostema diu[turnum] in pre[dicitis] lo[cis] in
pus conver[tetur]: oportet te esse attentum et cetera.
Artifex ydoneus tripplicem considerationem insinuat
in apostematibus secundum formam apostematis, secundum rupturam et secundum saniem. Et primo
secundum formam apostematis que sit laudabilis vel
que vituperanda. Si vero apostema emineat materia

---

[47] *fortasse* pernicitorias *vice* pernicatorias
[48] LX *emendum* XL
[49] *in* ad apostema sed, ad *redundans*

[50] *fortasse* suspiciosum *vice* suspicioso
[51] *fortasse* mutabile *vice* mutabili
[52] omnibus hijs elongatius est fluxus sanguinis de naribus *Vat 40rB*
[53] LX *Vat 40rB*

posita est exterius et non carni inviscata, ideo extra,
per quod declaratur quod caro non sit lesa et per
acutum propter fortitudinem caloris naturalis, habendo enim motum de centro incipit a diffusione latitudinis et protendit in acutum. Huius forma bona
est; ruptura apostematis laudabilis hec est ut materia
extra rumpatur et non intus. Intus enim si rumpatur
pessimum est quia membrum exterius putrefacit et
medicina apposita non bene consequatur suum effectum prius vim suam amittunt;[54] si enim rumpatur
extra bonum quia materia non inviscata carni, ut caro
ledatur, et medicina melius possunt[55] operari. Putredo laudatur si sit alba, quia declaratur materia non
esse cruda sed digesta et equalis per totum propter
abscentiam ventositatis, et hoc est quod dicit.

14. *Oportet ergo te esse attentum in hiis que compu-*
[*truerunt*], id est, que parabantur[56] ad putredinem.
Secundum huius[*modi*] *disciplinam*, quam dabimus,
quod emi[*net*] *et non est extra:*[57] quia materia carni inviscata[58] [*est*], *et pro*[*tendit*], id est, *intus minus:* quia
nichil eius apostematis interius est per quod declararatur[59] suspictio alterius apostematis interioris. *Et*
peracu[*tum*] *lau*[*dabile*]: hoc ascribitur caloris forti-
tudini que incipit a diffusione latitudinis et protendit
in acutum; si non esset acutum debilitas caloris declaretur unde mortificationem ostenderet. *Quod*
(129vA) *vero spa*[*ciosum*] *est:* ex hoc quod materia
carni est inviscata, unde putrefacit et carnem corrumpit. *Et mi*[*nime*] *ac*[*utum*] *pes*[*simum*]: quod declarat inbeccillitatem naturalis caloris non potentis
consequi proprium motum, incipientis a diffusione latitudinis et protendentis in acutum, et si calor est debilis mortificationem nature insinuat. *Eorum autem*
qui intus crepu[*erunt*] *siqua quidem exterius appa-*
[*ruerunt*] *pessimum:* quasi diceret quod si apostema
intus crepuerit et extra, ex eo quod apostema est intus
et extra, hoc provenit ex multo humore collecto ad
apostema quod sui presentia dissipando interiorem
partem dissipat exteriorem. *Quorum nil sani extra:*[60]
extra *bo*[*num*] *est:* ac si dicatur si materia colligatur
extra et apparet aliquod signum corruptionis bonum
est. *Quorum nil significat mali extra bonum est:* quia
non malum sed bonum indicat. Et *putre*[*do*] *ea*
lau[*datur*] *que est al*[*ba*]: ex diutina fortitudine caloris
materia vertitur in putredinem, et *equaliter per totum*,
quod non sit scrupulosa pro inbeccillitate caloris, *et in*
superificie equalis, propter abscentiam ventositatis,
neque mali odoris: neque fetidi neque gravis, quia
fetidus declarat corruptionem hu[*morum*] gravis
membrorum. *Que vero contraria pessima:* quia sicut
laudanda laudantur sic vituperanda vituperantur
propter corruptionem humorum et membrorum.

---

[54] *fortasse* amittit *vice* amittunt
[55] *fortasse* possit *vice* possunt
[56] peralbantur *Vat 40rB*
[57] omnino est extra *Vat 40rB*
[58] materia non inviscata carni *Vat 40rB*
[59] *fortasse* declaratur *vice* declararatur
[60] signum extra *vice* sani extra *Vat 40vA*

PARTICULA SECUNDA

15. [*Prognostics* VIII] *Omnis ydrops et cetera:* hic
secunde particule est principium quam ascribimus
virtuti naturali eo quod signa hic posita sumuntur
secundum vigorem vel vitium virtutis naturalis.
Inchoat enim ab ydropisi que habet provenire ex
errore virtutis epatis digestive. Videndum est ergo
quid sit ydropisis, quot sint eius species, ex quibus
causis habeant provenire, que sint earum curabiles et
que incurabiles et quarum[61] hee curabiles et incurabiles. Ydropisis sic describitur a G[aleno] in Passion-
ario: ydro[pisis] est error virtutis digestive epatis;
et a C[onstantino] in Viatico: ydro[pisis] est errare
virtu[tem] epatis digestivam. Huius descriptiones
dantur per causam, non enim ydropisis est error
(129vB) sed ex errore virtutis epatis digestive habet
provenire. Vel ydropisis est tumor vel inflatio membrorum innaturalis ex errore virtutis epatis digestive
provenientis.[62] Dum dicitur tumor due species denotantur, scilicet, leucoflegmantia, ypo[sarca] vel
ana[sarca], quare humor est causa et humoris est
tumorem operari. Dum dicitur inflatio due alie
species denotantur, scilicet, timpanites et asclites,
quare ventositas est causa et ventositatis est infla-
tionem operari. Sunt autem quattuor species ydropisis: leucoflegmantia, anasarca vel ypo[sarca], timpanites et asclites. Leuco[flegmantia] dicitur a
leucoë quod album est, et flegmantia, flegma, eo quod
haec species ydropisis fit de albo flegmate, scilicet
naturali. Ypo[sarca] dicitur ab ypos quod est sub
et sarcos, caro, eo quod in hac specie ydropisis materia
sit posita sub carne. Anasarca dicitur ab ana quod
est iuxta et sarcos, caro, quod in hac specie sit posita
iuxta carnem materia. Timpanites dicitur a timpano
eo quod venter eorum repercussus resonat in modum
timpani. Asclites dicitur [ab ἀσκός quod est] venter
eo quod venter talium consistat ut venter semiplenus.
Leucoflegmantia [habet fieri] ex distemperantia universali epatis in frigiditate et humiditate quasi
potentialibus. Ana[sarca] habet fieri ex universali
distemperantia epatis in frigiditate et siccitate quasi
potentialibus. Timpanites fit ex distemperantia gibbi
epatis in caliditate et siccitate quasi potentialibus,
syme vero in frigiditate. Asclites habet fieri ex distemperantia gibbi in caliditate et humiditate quasi
potentialibus, syme vero in frigiditate, quod sic
attendendum est. Dum universaliter epar distemperatur in frigiditate et humiditate fit indigestio; ex
indigestione per frigiditatem et humiditatem proveniente, multa flegmatici humoris fit generatio; per
frigiditatem constringentem et humiditatem lubri-
cantem sequitur vigor virtu[tis] expul[sive]. Humor
ergo generatus venatim mittitur per universum corpus,
unde tumorem prestat in intrinsecis corporis partibus
et inducitur quedam species ydropisis que dicitur

---

[61] *fortasse* quare *vice* quarum
[62] *fortasse* proveniens *vice* provenientis

leucoflegmantia. Dum universaliter epar distemperatur in frigiditate et siccitate quasi potentialibus, (130rA) fit indigestio, ex indigestione proveniente per frigiditatem constringentem et siccitatem intercidentem multa superfluorum fit generatio; per frigiditatem constringentem sequitur vigor virtutis expulsive, per siccitatem intercidentem agentem in superflua operatur ad generationem ventositatis, unde superflua generata ex vigore virtutis expulsive et per ventositatem illa generata impellentem tumorem operatur et ventositas quia crossa est non potest exire dum querit exitum et non potest conculcatur et corrumpitur, unde inducit fetorem et hec species dicitur yposarcha vel anasarca. Interdum sequitur distemperantiam gibbi in caliditate et siccitate; per caliditatem dissolventem fit apertio pororum, unde spiritus et humores exalant asmia, per poros apertos fit qualis infrig[i]datio sime unde per frigiditatem prepedientem digestionem plurima adiuvantur superflua unde per caliditatem dissolvuntur; per siccitatem intercidentem plurima fit generatio ventositas cuius ventositatis sequitur interclusio inter gibbum et sifac, ventositatis non potest exire per alia membra propter vigorem virtutis epatis attractive et sic ventositas illa inflat ventrem et hec species dicitur timpanites. Interdum sequitur distemperantia gibbi in caliditate et humiditate, per calorem fit proorum apertio, spiritus et hu[mores] exalant asyma et emittuntur per poros apertos unde sima infrig[i]datur, per humiditatem fit multa generatio superfluorum coöperante caliditate gibbi et liquorosa sunt superflua, et per caliditatem dissolventem fit generatio ventositatis, hec omnia inter zirbum et sifac inflant et fit asclites. Speciebus ydropisis sufficienter assignatis videndum est quibus ex causis ydropisis habeat provenire. Ydropisis est error virtutis aut provenit vitio epatis principaliter aut principali vitio intestinorum aut principali vitio stomachi aut principali vitio spiritualium aut principali (130rB) vitio splenis aut principali vitio renum aut ex nimia sanguinis effusione aut per retentionem eiusdem. Principali vitio epatis fit ydropisis sicut ex premissis potest intelligi vel fit alio modo principali vitio epatis propter apostema in epate exortum ex quo apostemate intantum debilitatur epatis natura quod non potest digerere ptisanariam sucositatem illuc transmissam et sic prepeditur digestio et sic ydropisis. Vitio stomachi habet fieri, nam virtus membrorum cuiuslibet prefixum et determinatum habet terminum ut actionem suam perficiat et alterius perficere nequid,[63] unde impossibile est terciam digestionem omnium membrorum bonam fieri nisi bona fiat in stomacho. Epar per suam naturem non potest supplere quod defuit in stomacho unde cum mala celebratur digestio in epate fit indigestio et sic ydropisis provenit. Vitio intestinorum vel ex retentione fecum propter constipationem vel propter inmoderatum fluxum intestinorum, propter constipationem dum

feces nequeunt exire, dum enim attrahitur succositas ptisanaria ad epar attrahuntur feces inmixte succositati unde corrumpunt sucositatem et calor conculcatur et prepeditur digestio fitque indigestio et sic ydropisis. Ex nimio fluxu intestinorum, nam dum ptisanaria sucositas mittitur ad intestina propter fluxum effluit per intestina unde dum non mittitur ad epar ad refocilandum calorem naturalem epatis quia ab humiditate rei ptisanarie debet calor foveri, unde dum eius non invenit fomentum ocultatur unde contrarie qualitatis consurgit effectus, scilicet frigiditatis, unde per frigiditatem prepeditur digestio fitque indigestio et sic ydropisis. Vitio spiritualium dum enim spiritualia disponuntur in nimia caliditate et siccitate sitis provenit propter exsiccationem oris stomachi unde aquam assumit in multa quantitate ex aqua prepeditur prima digestio. Si prima digestio est mala secunda erit mala, unde consurgit ydrops. Vel quia caliditate et siccitate viget virtus attractiva in spiritualibus unde (130vA) trahunt per ramum vene concave. Vena concava sugit a venis capillaribus sucositatem epatis inexcoctam unde prepeditur digestio, fit indigestio et sic ydropisis. Vitio splenis vel ex oppilatione simul ex repletione sui comprimente epar dum oppilatur splen non potest recipere melancolicam materiam quia eius est expurgamentum remanet in epate, sui frigiditate debilitat epar et utraque qualitas operatur defectionem digestionis unde fit indigestio et sic ydropisis. Iterum dum comprimitur epar ex splene turgido sucositas non potest digeri fit indigestio et ydropisis. Vitio renum dum viget virtus attractiva in renibus ut in diabete trahunt illam sucositatem inexcoctam, color[64] obtunditur et contrarie qualitatis vigor sequitur scilicet frigiditatis, fit indigestio et ydropisis; ex fluxu sanguinis provenit quia sanguis est fomentum caloris deficiente[65] sanguine et calor[e] unde fit prepeditur digestio et sic ydropisis; ex retentione, dum sanguis retinetur et redundat ad epar debilitat epar et fit indigestio et sic ydropisis. Videndum est que species ydropisis sunt curabiles et que incurabiles, id est, difficiles ad curandum. Curabiles ut leucoflegmantia et ana[sarca] vel ypo[sarca], difficiles ad curandum timpanites et asclites. Merito lecuoflegmantia et ana[sarca] vel ypo[sarca] sunt curabiles quia fiunt ex universali distemperantia epatis ut leucoflegmantia ex naturali distemperantia epatis in frigiditate et humiditate. Anasarca fit ex universali distemperantia in frigiditate et siccitate et quia contraria contrariis curantur, contraria utrique morbo distemperata in contraria qualitate possunt exhiberi ducendo corpus ad sanitatem. Ut calida et sicca laboranti leucoflegmantia, calida et humida laboranti anasarca vel yposarca; vel alio modo iudicantur curabiles quia medicamen sumptum in corpore iuvatur a virtutibus, et virtus expulsiva fortis est in utraque

---

[63] *fortasse* nequeat *vice* nequid

[64] *fortasse* calor *vice* color
[65] calor deficiat unde prepeditur digestio *Vat 41rA*

quare iuvat medicamen in educatione[m][66] malorum humorum (130vB) ex quibus provenit ydropisis. Iterum alia est causa, quia he species fiunt ex humore unde medicina inveniens coherentiam in humore in re solida, medicina processu temporis consequitur quidem suum est[67] et sic educto humore egritudo cessat. Iterum e contrario alie sunt difficiles ad curandum propter dissonam distemperantiam qualitatum in utrisque. Tympanites fit ex distemperantia gibbi in caliditate et siccitate, syme vero in frigiditate. Calida non possunt dari propter distemperantiam gibbi in caliditate quia omne simile suum simile augmentat et facit furere, frigida propter distemperantiam syme in frigiditate non possunt dari, temperata minime, quia omne minus violentum a magis violento permutatur et cetera. Iterum medicina supscepta a virtute explusiva non adiuvatur quia fiunt ex defectu virtu[tis] expulsive. Iterum hec species habent copiam ventositatis unde medicina non invenit coherentiam in re subtili et aërea et sic non potest illa ventositas expelli, ipsa vero medicina operatur ad maiorem ventositatis generationem et sic fit error peior priore.

16. *Omnis ydrops in acuta egri[tudine malum]* et *cetera:* videtur plane contrarium quomodo ydropisis possit supervenire in acuta egritudine cum feb[re], sit morbus [realis][68] calidus et sit calor accidentalis. Ydropisis sit morbus frigidus, solutione dictus quid[69] hydropisis est morbus frigidus quasi potentialis, febris est morbus calidus quasi actualis. Morbus calidus vero quasi actualis non est contrarius frigiditati quasi potentiali. *Vere omnis ydrops in acuta egri[tudine] ma[lum] est:* quia febris morbus calidus ydrops morbus frigidus calida non possunt exhibere pro febre, frigida pro ydropisi, temperata minime. *Infestatur enim fe[bre] g[ravedine] et do[lore]:* per hoc vult auctor notare quod malum sit si ydrops fuerit cum febre, quia fe[bris] morbus est consimilis unde natura consimilium est immutata. Malum est si fit cum gravedine cum proveniat ex repletione unde est enim morbus officialis factus vitio forme unde natura officialis est im(131rA)mutata, humor replens extendendo inducit solutionem continuitatis, unde malum est si sit dolor, quia natura utroque est mutata, ergo phisis composita ex omnibus virtutibus non potest resistere morbo neque per naturam consimilium neque per naturam offi[cialum][70] neque per naturam utrorumque. Et *ideo ydrops cum febre malum consurgit aut[em] ex lumbis et yliis:* auctor intendit assignare unde ydrops habeat provenire, provenit ex lumbis ut ipse testatur, hoc est, ex renibus. Renes namque effecti sitibundi, ut est videri in diabete, attrahunt sucositatem ptisanariam inexcoctam quare prepeditur secunda di-

gestio et fit indigestio [et] ydropisis vitio renum. Ylia dicuntur intestina, ponit autem partem pro toto, vel provenit propter constipationem vel propter fluxum, ut dictum est, vel quandoque provenit vitio subtilis intestini ubi ventositas intercluditur et fit strophus. In talibus intestinis resident interius unde fit constipatio, superfluitates prime digestionis mittuntur ad epar et corrumpunt ptisanarium sucositatem a qua mala celebratur digestio secunda unde provenit ydro[ps]. *Est et ab epate*, id est, que species fit principali vitio epatis ydro[ps] consurgit ab epate vel ex natural[i] distemperantia epatis in frigiditate et humiditate vel frigiditate et siccitate vel ex distemperantia gibbi in caliditate et humiditate, syme in frigiditate quasi potentialibus. Vel ex apostemate, *consurgens aut ex lumbis*, id est, renibus et yliis, id est, intestinis *significatur ex pe[dum] infl[atione]*. Nam dum fit vitio intestinorum hoc provenit dum fit constipatio in intestinis, attrahitur subductio inmoderate ad epar, unde epar debilitatur, calor accidentalis consurgens ex indigestione ventositatem generat crossam, crosse ille fumositates per tertium ramum quilis vene mittuntur ad inferiora mediantibus venis saphenis quare fit pedis inflatio. Et *ventris diuturna effusione:* huius ydropisis com[m]itatur nimiam effusionem ventris, hoc est, effusionem vene per virgam; (131rB) venter duo habet expurgamenta, unum per pudicum circulum alterum per virgam et huius effusio fit per virgam quia renes sitibundi attrahendo in multa quantitate illam sucositatem quare multum emittitur per virgam. *Non tamen cum de[fectu] do[loris]:* pungenti non facti[71] ex humore sed ex ventositate extendente; *se[u] ven[tris] tu[morem]*, propter multam ventositatem in ventre pariter cum humore operante tumorem. *Cuius origo est ab epate:* scilicet si proveniat vitio epatis, *fit ut tussicula:* quia ex quacumque causa proveniat ex vitio epatis facta principaliter adest cum tussicula, si fiat ex universali distemperantia, vel ex distemperantia gibbi, vel ex apostemate nam dum plurima congeries hu[morum] est in epate coadunata epar inflatur, comprimit stomachum, stomachus spiritualia, spiritualis traceam arteriam, quare fit offendiculum spiritus in traceam arteriam et fit tussis; *nec quicquam proiciunt:* quia non est materia in spiritualibus, et *pe[des] tument*, propter multam ventositatem que inmittitur ad pedes per tercium ramum quilis vene. Et *non egerunt nisi mo[dicum]:* propter defectum virtutis explusive, unde retinentur feces et constipant et hoc locum habet in timpanite, et *cum angustia*, quia modicum est et durum. Et *circa ven[trem] apostema fiunt:* provenientia ex superfluitatibus generatis per indigestionem, et non proprie sunt fumositates intercluse inflantes in modum apostematum. Et *non continuo extra manantia:* quia cum crosse sunt fumositates non cotidie possunt excludi per poros; *sed quandoque veluti fu[gientia]:* quia fumositatum non est habere pre-

---

[66] ad eductionem *Vat 41rA*
[67] *fortasse* effectum *vice* est
[68] morbus realis *Vat 41rA*
[69] *fortasse* quod *vice* quid
[70] officialium *Vat 41rB*

[71] *fortasse* pungens non factus *vice* pungenti non facti

fixum locum. [*Prognostics* IX] *Si caput et plante manuum et pe[dum][72] fri[gide] fu[erint]*: in febre acuta dum ydropisis malum frigiditas extremitatum malum nunciat vel hoc provenit propter defectum naturalis caloris vel propter defectum nutrimenti;[73] quia dum fit indigestio deficit nutrimentum unde deficit calor propter defectum pabuli sicut humor naturalis nutrimentum est corporis sicut (132vA) pabulum corporis quod patet mollito. Et *venter et latera et mandibule ca[luerint] malum est:* propter indigestionem calor accidentalis consurgens ventrem calefacit et propter collimitantiam calent mandibule. *Bo[num] est egrum ex toto calere*: quia non est defectus caloris naturalis neque nutrimenti adest defectus, et *mollem ac suavem convenienter esse:* non habere cutis asperitatem propter defectum siccitatis exasperantis. Naturalis mollities bona est quia defectum insinuat siccitatis consumentis humiditatem. *Bonum est mo[deste] et id est non laboriose et rep[ente] eundem [vi]deatur:*[74] propter defectum superflui humoris aggravantis non enim adest humor aggravans unde levis videatur. *Gravis vero si fuerit:* vel propter humores aggravantes vel propter defectum spiritum, *manus quoque et pe[des] pon[derosa]:* propter humorem adgravantem vel propter defectum spirituum iam virtus regitiva nequid regere membra in proprio scemate et propria positione, *orrendum est:* talia enim signa mortem sunt minantia. *Si vero livor:* proveniens per frigiditatem operantem indigestionem unde frigiditas operans indigestionem a re indigesta aqueam humiditatem exprimit, ut est videri in torculari, unde terrestris efficitur res indigesta talis res indigesta ungues digitorum inficit secundum livorem. *Unguibus digitisque admixtis videri:*[75] quo ad materiam referatur quia materia generata per frigiditatem mortificantem admiscetur rei generate per calorem adurentem. *Mortem adventare non dubi[tabis]:* multa fuit materia frigida et calida et per calidam materiam facta est adustio in corde deputato ad vitam. *Quod si livor*, id est, terrestritas proveniens per calorem consumentem subtilia unde terrestria remanent ex parte; *admixtus viridi*, per admixtionem terrestrium et ignearum parcium fit viridis color. *Si vero his ungues non infec[erit]*, id est, si non apparuerit in unguibus non est succensio in spiritualibus (131vB) que possit operari ad unguium viriditatem, licet hoc est quam vix viriditas. *Cetera corri[puerit]*, id est, infecerit quia provenit talis viriditas ab epate et non a corde deputato, *spei locus*, id est, salutis, *non deerit.* Non enim viriditas prorumpens ab epate proveniet ex tanta furiositate materie sicut lividitas prorumpens a corde hoc signum provenit in sinthomatis quia ex

cordis furore illud vero vi[riditas] quod fit ab epate potentis se exhonerare a superfluis.

17. *Proderit et cetera:* dixerat auctor superius quod viridis color in unguibus mortem declarabit propter succensionem factam in membro deputato ad vitam, sed notandum quod ante viridis color est in unguibus et adest facilis action inspirandi et respirandi que declarat bonam cordis dispositionem et ideo mortem non insinuat, et hoc est quod dicit. *Proderit cuncta signa perpen[dere]*, investigare signa salutifera et mortifera ut sciamus iudicare de futura morte vel vita. *Quod si egrum viridis*[76] *suffi[cienter]:* ut modo bene valeat tolerare, et *una bo[ni] significatio affuerit*, id est, actio inspirandi et respirandi que per Anthonium Musam[77] dicitur bona, *terminus tibi promittitur salutis*, id est, talis determinatio ad salutem habet fieri quasi diceret ista duo signa sunt meliora in egritudine, fortitudo infirmi morbum suum tolerare et cetera, facilis actio inspirandi et respirandi. *Cum quolibet exteriori apostemate*, sive proveniat ex materia furiosa sive cruda, *sed palloris*[78] *predicti loci pericula non deerunt*, id est, infectio in predictis locis in unguibus, scilicet adducit periculum materia furiosa, dissipando ungues facit ipsos cadere.

18. *Si testes et virga et cetera:* circa dispositionem testiculorum pariter et virge actoris est intentio pronosticari et in febribus acutis ex horum dispositione future mortis vel vite eliciuntur pronostica. (132rA) Ad horum membrorum consistentiam copia mittitur nervorum, venarum et arteriarum et spirituum in prima generatione animalis masculini sexus et ad virge generationem de substantia venarum et arteriarum et nervorum conveniunt. In essentiam unius substantie uniuntur et quoddam membrum offitiale consistunt quod adiacet virge a parte subteriori, unde spiritus animalis illuc mittitur vitalis et naturalis et inflat membrum illud unde virga inflatur. Si vero diminui videatur virga, aut provenit hoc ex defectu spirituum, ut est videri in spasmo ex inanitione ubi fit spirituum defectus, aut provenit ex apostemate exorto in principali membro. Dum enim aliquod apostema oritur in membro principali, testes et virga ut membra exposita et exteriora mittunt spiritum et calorem coadiuvamentum membri nobilis, spiritibus deficientibus inflantibus virgam, virga videtur minui et hoc est quod dicit; *si testes et virga ultra so[litum] minui*, ut talis diminutio sit innaturalis, *contrahique appa[ruerit]*, ex contractione nervorum contrahuntur membra quibus sunt alligati et talis contractio provenit ex consumptione substantialis humiditatis et indicat spasmum ex inanitione. *Aut ni[mium] do[loris] aut mor[tis] adven[tum] pronun[ciabis]:* huius namque diminutio indicat apostema, contractio spasmum indicat ex inanitione qui incurabilis est, per calorem namque adurentem fit consumptio

---

[72] Si capud et plante pedum et vole manuum *Vat 41vB* frigide fuerint

[73] nutrimenti *notatum delendi est a scriba*

[74] Bonum est et modeste et non laboriose et non repente in eadem laterum commutare *Vat 41rA*

[75] *fortasse* viridi *vice* videri

[76] videris *Vat 41vA*

[77] Antonio Masice *Vat 41vA*

[78] *fortasse* caloris *vice* palloris

humorum et deperditio spirituum quibus anima corpori est irretita, hiis deperditis anima a corde sequestratur unde mors.

19. [*Prognostics* X] *Sompnus vero moris est conveniens:* omnis significatio aut sumitur ex forma corporis aut ex actionibus aut ex superfluitatibus. Postquam auctor posuit signa que sumuntur ex forma corporis nunc intendit ponere signa que sumuntur ex actionibus et ideo circa sompni dispositionem intendit pronosticari. Sompnus est quies animalium (132rB) virtutum cum intensione naturalium, id est, in sompno animales virtutes quiescunt, licet non omnes sed proprie virtus visibilis dicitur quiescere. Intenduntur naturales appetitus di[gestio], re[gestio et] ex[pulsio]: et cibis et potibus per triplicem digestionem, digestis multiplex resolvitur fumositas que cerebrum petit tanquam tocius corporis caminum; eius relaxando miringas et humectando comprimunt cerebrum, coangustatur in suis meatibus unde parum debilitatur, dilatatur et constringitur. Per angustos meatus spiritus visibilis non mittitur ad oculos ut excitet virtu[tem] animalem visibilem unde sompnus inducitur. Calor enim in nocte revocatur ad interiora, in die non, quia anima vacat extrinsecas perficere actiones vel operationes, quo multiplicato interius hu[mores] extenuat, spiritus crossos subtiliat quia spiritus sunt instrumenta virtu[tum] et spiritus subtilitati melius excitant virtu[tes] ad suas actiones perficiendas. Calor ipse naturalis multiplicatus virtutes vivificat et sic virtu[tes] animales intenduntur. Merito dicitur sompnus est quies animalium virtutum et cetera. Sompnus multipliciter consideratur in quantitate, qualitate et tempore. In quantitate quia aut multus aut paucus aut mediocris. Multus aut fit ex multitudine ciborum et potuum a quibus multa resolvitur fumositas, aut fit ex multa humiditate praehibente in cerebro ubi est videri in litargia propter oppilationem ventriculorum cerebri, dum spiritus nequeat venire per continuitatem meatuum ad oculos. Falsus sompnus inducitur aut provenit ex mortificatione, ut est videri in acceptione opii. Paucus sompnus fit vel ex paucitate cibo[rum] et po[tuum] vel ex cerebri siccitate ut in frenesi vel ex dolore quia omnis dolor exacuit reuma et ad locum dolentem confluunt hu[mores] dissecantes[79] et pungentes. In qualitate consideratur, quia aut suavis aut insuavis. Suavis sompnus bonam dispositionem cerebri insinuat et panniculorum eius, insuavis malam dispositionem (132vA) cerebri insinuat et panniculorum eius. In tempore consideratur quia naturale tempus sompni est nox. Obscuritas visus congregativa sicut claritas disgregativa, frigiditas noctis est reductiva caloris ad intrinseca; inducto ca[lore] ad intrinseca dissolvit fumositates et sompnum inducit. Naturale tempus vigiliarum est dies, quia claritas est visus disgregativa et dum animal[80] vacat extrinsecas perficere actiones

vigiliarum instantia sequitur. Sompnus qui fit a mane usque ad tertiam non est vituperandus quia tunc sunt hore sanguinis, et ex sanguine mulcebris resolvitur fumositas que sompnum inducit; littera plana est.

20. [*Prognostics* X] *Stercoris egestio et cetera:* positis signis que sumuntur ex forma corporis [et] ex actionibus eius secundum proprietatem virtu[tis] digestive nunc intendit ponere signa que sumuntur ex superfluitatibus secundum proprietatem [virtutis] digestivam,[81] et primo pronosticatur circa superfluitatem prime digestionis que proprie dicitur subudctio et pronosticatur circa eam: primo in eo quod est mala, [...] quarto in eo quod est peior, quinto in eo quod est pessima. Subductio multipliciter consideratur, in quantitate, qualitate, tempore, numero, tenuitate et spissitudine et modo exitus. In quantitate quia aut multa aut pauca aut mediocris et tam multa quam pauca aut fit vi nature aut fit vi sinthomatis. Multa fit vi nature, quando natura bene digestam et divisam materiam per secessum evacuat, ita tamen quod ex hac eductione eger suavior et levior efficitur immo in salutem restituitur. Multa fit vi sinthomatis aut fit qualitate aut quantitate. Aut quantitate et qualitate aut ex membrorum incontinentia: qualitate tantum ut est videri in dissinteria, secundum quod in Glossulis Anfforismorum. Pauca fit vi nature quando natura bene digestam et divisam materiam per alias regiones evacuat, parum remanet in intestinis unde pauca subductio et ex tali eductione eger levior et suavior efficitur immo in salutem restituitur. Pauca fit vi sinthomatis ex acumine caloris transeuntis feces (132vB) in scybala et in maniam[82] ferri, secundum quod Galenus recitat de quodam constipato cui factum fuit clister et sentiebat intus, tandem insistebat Galenus cum unguentis mollificantibus et facta est relaxatio pudici circuli et emisit quasi ferream substantiam. De eodem recitat quod cum acciperet cibaria per vomitum emittebat. In qualitate consideratur in colore, odore, in tenuitate et spissitudine. In colore consideratur quia si fuerit subcitrina, media inter liquidam et solidam laudatur, significat enim temperantiam duorum humorum qui transmittuntur ad intestina et ad stomachum, scilicet flegmatis et colere. Flegma transmittitur ad stomachum ut iuvet[83] virtus expulsiva et de eo mittitur ad intestina ut lubricando iuvet[83] virtus expulsiva et feces educantur. Colera mittitur ad stomachum ut iuvet[83] virtus appetitiva et de ea mittitur ad intestina ut mordicando procuret ventris offitium. In egestione non prevalet flegmaticus humor ut sui albedine prestet album colorem, neque colera ut sui colorem citrinum

---

[79] *fortasse* dessicantes *vice* dissecantes
[80] *fortasse* anima *vice* animal, *vide* 19.17

[81] *post* digestivam *addit Vat 42rA:* primo auctor pronosticatur circa superfluitates prime digestionis que duplex est nam alia est crossa que vocatur subductio alia subtilis que unctuositas appelatur primo autem circam crossam superfluitatem prognosticatus que dicitur subductio que quadrupliciter consideratur.
[82] *fortasse* maneriem *vice* maniam
[83] *fortasse* iuvat *vice* iuvet

prestet sed ex utraque contradictione compositus color provenit, scilicet subcitrinus. Item significat temperantiam qualitatum activarum, scilicet frigiditatis et caliditatis, non enim prevalet caliditas ut inducat per adustionem nigrum colorem, neque frigiditas ut inducat album, sed ex utraque contradictione color compositus provenit; etiam significat temperamentum qualitatum passivarum, scilicet siccitatis et humiditatis. Non prevalet siccitas ut prestet duritiem per suum motum ad centrum neque humiditas ut relaxando reddat subductionem fluxilem sed alterutra contradictione media est inter liquidam et solidam. Iterum si fuerit citrini coloris significat coleram, si albi flegma, si rubri sanguinem, si lividi mortificationem, si viridis adustionem, si nigri aliquod precedentium. In odore si fetida ultra modum corruptionem humorum gravius[84] membrorum [declarat]; in tenuitate et spissitudine si fuerit tenuis et liquida subtilium humorum declarat habundantiam, si spissa solidorum. In tempore consideratur quia debet fieri in media nocte celebrata digestione vel iuxta consuetudinem. In numero consideratur quia si sepe emittitur per indigestionem fit et corpus male (133rA) nutritur. In modo exitus consideratur quia si fuerit cum sonitu vituperatur quia declarat debilitatem caloris non potentis consumere ventositatem factam per indigestionem. *Stercoris egestio:* quelibet superfluitas attestatur vigori vel vitio dispositionis membrorum in quibus generatur stercus namque seu alio nomine dicatur in stomacho et intestinis generatur unde attestatur vigori vel vitio dispositionis stomachi et intestinorum, dicit: *stercoris egestio*, id est, id quod per egestionem educitur stercus est; *si numque*[85] *exsiccata fu[erit]*, per quod declaratur abscentia siccitatis consumentis; *neque li[qiuda] omnino*, cum ventosiate pro defectu liquidorum humorum; *sed seiuncta*, id est, media inter liquidam et solidam. *Hora solita eve[nire]*, per quod declaratur quod corpus non est multum permutatum a priori consistentia. *Signum est ea que sunt sub diafragma est salubria liquida*, id est, non unctuosa. *Bona*, quia non emittitur pinguedo corporis per secessum. Pronosticatus est auctor circa perfectam egestionem, nunc intendit pronosticari circa minus bona[m] et vere liquida bona est per quod declaratur fortitudo caloris dissolventis unde liquida videtur egestio, non enim simpliciter bona est, *et si fuerit sine so[nitu]* ventoso, quia calor naturalis potestas fuit ad dissolvendum et consumendum superfluam ventositatem; *nec inordi[nate] malum*, ordo attenditur in egestione ut incipiat et sine sonitu desinat, inordinatum esset modo cum sonitu postea sine sonitu. *Si enim fre[quenter] malum:* cum quadam frequenti emissione que fluxus dicitur *ma[ximo] la[bore] af[ficitur] eger:* laboriosum est admodum patientem inconstanter assellare pro fluxu immoderato fit deperditio spirituum et humorum unde debitum

nutrimentum non subministratur membris nutriendis et *vigiliis*, pro defectu nutrimenti qui provenit ex fluxu pauperato corpore nutrimento, siccitas innascitur unde sequitur vigiliarum instantia. Et *in defectum adducit* patientem dum fit deperdito vinculorum quibus anima corpori est irretita. *Utile est stercus secundum quantitatem assumptorum evenire:* ut si multa sint as(133rB)sumpta multa subductio. Iterum dicendum si multa sint cibaria affinia humane nature que attrahantur a membris unde pauca subductio, vel sint alia cibaria que sunt inimica naturis et si pauca sint multa erit subductio et *bis vel ter in die*, in die enim non celebratur perfecta digestio, unde superflua generata in die bis vel ter educuntur. *In nocte semel*, quia in nocte celebrata perfecta digestione non multa generantur sed que generantur semel sunt educenda, et *luce proxima*, quia tunc sunt hore sanguinis inde tunc temporis a sanguine quedam resolvitur fumositas que virtutes naturales iuvat quare tunc competens fit explusio. *Aut so[lito] mo[re] contin[gere]:* per quod declaratur quod natura plurimum defatigata unde iam istud retine[t] consuetudinem et consuetudo est secunda natura. *Utile est etiam appropin[quante] termino egritudinis*, solutionis, *idem stercus densari*, ut sit simplex relatio et personalis, id est, mediocritatem habere cum densitate per quod declaratur contemperamentum qualitatum passivarum, scilicet, siccitatis et humiditatis; et *[si] co[loris] subci[trini] fu[erit]:*[86] hic color declarat moderantiam humorum colere et flegmatis et temperantiam istarum qualitatum frigiditatis et caliditatis. Ne aliquis intelligat quod stercus densetur in solidum, ideo dicit *nec in solido condempsari*, quia si esset condempsatum in solidum declaret fortem calorem adurentem.

21. *Bonum est si lumbricos admixtos habuerit:* fortis enim calor naturalis qui potest humores in animalia transmutare. Calor enim agens in humores superficietenus eos obvolvit crustula ut panis in clibano. Caliditas potentialis cum calore accidentali latens interius dissolvit in fumositates, quia plenius dissolute maiorem suscipiunt subtilitatem et fit generatio spiritus naturalis. Ipse spiritus querit exitum, non potest exire suppositione crustule et fit generatio lumbrici. Lumbrici generatio fit ex speciebus flegmatis; ex colera non fit quia amara necant lumbricos; ex melancolia non quia habet qualitates mortificatorias; ex sanguine non quia ut dicit auctor si sanguis in ventrem effu(133vA)nditur praeter naturam in saniem convertitur. Generatio autem aut fit ex flegmate salso et sunt longi et rotundi per caliditatem elongantem, rotundi per siccitatem rotundantem; ex flegmate dulci sunt longi et lati, longi per caliditatem elongantem, lati per humiditatem diffusionem latitudinis operantem; et isti pessimi sunt, habentes istos in utero putant habere serpentes. Aut fuerit ex flegmate acerbo et sunt breves et rotundi: breves per

---

[84] *fortasse* gravium *vice* gravius
[85] *fortasse* neque *vice* numque

[86] et colore subcitrino fieri *Vat 42vA*

frigiditatem incurtantem, rotundi per siccitatem rotundantem; ex flegmate naturali breves et lati: breves per frigiditatem incurtantem, lati per humiditatem diffundentem. Sumunt plerumque formas a loco secundum dispositionem intestinorum, quidam generantur in ieiuno, quidam in gracilibus intestinis, et hoc alibi insinuatur.

22. *In omni acu[ta] egritudine non vent[rem] ple[num]*, id est, a malis habentibus[87] non sit repletum, sed ut *vacui*, id est, a malis humoribus sit evacuatum, sed aliquis posset intelligere de evacuatione que sit pro defectu carnis, dicit *non te[nuem]*, id est, maceratum, *sed carnosum*, secundum propriam formam. *In ve[ntrem] bo[num] est aquosum vero stercus et id est liquidum:* quod declarat indigestionem et subtilium humorum habundantiam, id est, in quos humores medicina data non invenit coherentiam, sed quia posset esse liquidum colericum vel melancolicum quia licet quidam humores sint sicci, quidam humidi, omnes in substantia humorosi. Ideo dicit *sive album*, quod declarat frigiditatem facientem summam et ultimam indigestionem, quia sicut urina alba significat ultimam indigestionem, sic et stercus talis coloris, *aut nimis citri[num]*, quod significat principium adustionis, *vel spumosum malum est:* Omnis spuma cum colore significante calorem furoris est inditium, sed cum colore significante frigiditatem indigestionem vel ventositatis admixitionem insinuat. *Item mo[dicum] malum est:* hoc contingit quando natura parum laborat in extremis partibus pro mortificatione, et *viscosum*, per siccitatem inserentem et leve, id est, fluidum, *sive album*, ex indigestione, *sive citrinum*, ex calore adurente, (133vB) *aut spumosum*, propter ebullitionem. *Pessimum et mortis signum nigrum:* niger color aut significat adustionem aut mortificationem, ex precedenti viridi adustionem, ex precedenti livido mortificationem, et *fetidum*, corruptionem humoris, et *viride*, primum adustionis. *Varium*, id est, varii co[lores] longi[88] egri[tudinis] quia multus est humor in causa, *neque minus signum est mortis*, id est, ita est pernitiosum et mortale, *quam istud stercus quod profert loturam intestinorum:* quod apparet in prima specie dissinterie; et *colorem porrorum*. Si fuerit pernitiosus est propter adustionem materie prassina colera est in causa, *sive nigrum malum*, predicta ratione. *Contingit etiam isotos colores simul evenire:* quoniam multi humores sunt in causa et tunc pessimum est; color enim viridis si per se fuerit malum nunciat, *quod si fuerit* cum nigro colore, citrino et albo [pessimum].

23. *Ventositas et cetera:* auctor circa crossam superfluitatem prime digestionis que dicitur subductio est pronosticatus, nunc intendit pronosticari circa superfluitatem prime digestionis subtilem que dicitur ventositas. Superfluitas prime digestionis aut grossa aut subtilis, calor aut fortis aut debilis, debilis calor agens in subtilem superfluitatem eam sufficit dissolvere et

resolvere sed non extenuare. Dissoluta superfluitas querit exitum, obviat aëri extrinseco, unde ex alterutra allisione et quod fit ei exitus per angustum sonat. Item fortis calor agens in crossam superfluitatem ipsam dissolvit et plurimum in subtiles superfluitates transducit que querunt exitum et obviat aëri et sic exit cum sonitu. Calor mediocris agens in grossam superfluitatem tantum dissolvit quantum sufficit consumere, materiam in mediocrem grossitiem transducit, sed natura superfluitatis a mediocri calore dissoluta exit sine sonitu. Quare melior ventositas sine sonitu pro mediocri actione caloris quam illa que est cum sonitu aut declarat (134rA) fortitudinem caloris aut debil[itat]em ut dictum. *Vento[sitas] sine so[nitu] la[udabilis]:* intelligas quam illa que est cum sonitu et *illa que est cum so[nitu] me[lior] est quam que interclusa:* retenta enim fumositas petit exitum, non potest per inferiora educi, rapitur ad superiora et admixta spiritibus libere non possunt, mitti per cerebrum aggravatur cerebrum et in suis actionibus ebatur. *Significat amentem:* vera fit amentia extendendo aliquam partem et solvendo continuitatem inducit dolorem. *Aut do[lorem] la[borantem] nisi sit vo[luntarie]* retenta, scilicet ut cum aliquis conversatur inter probos et non potest eam emittere unde voluntarie retinetur et quia aliquociens reddit ad ypocondria et inducit dolorem. In ipsis ideo dicit *do[lor] in ypo[condriis] hanc* proprietatem habet, id est, naturam, *si recens fu[erit]*, id est, de novo adveniens ut sit ex ventositate et *sine calore*, ad maiorem certitudinem quod non sit ex materia calida et removetur materia sine [sonitu]; dicit recens quia materia frigida recens dolorem non inducit sed durabilem. *Si ru[gitus] super[venerit]:* quia praeco est ventositatis unde iam materia movetur ad exitum, et *cum egestione*, hoc est, per secessum, quia redundat materia, illa quandoque per secessum quandoque per urinam solvitur. Venter enim duo habet expurgamenta: aut per secessum aut per urinam, sed contingit quandoque quod talis ventositas veniens ad ventrem neque per secessum neque per ventrem emittitur, sed veniendo ad oxeum inflat unde videntur crivosi et non sunt, aut descendit per tercium ramum quilis vene ad pedes et inflat ipsos et videntur ydropici et non sunt: *alioquin ad inferiora transmutantur.*

24. [*Prognostics* XII] *Urina laudabilis et cetera:* circa dupplicem superfluitatem prime digestionis auctor est pronosticatus, scilicet circa crossam et subtilem. Nunc communiter intendit pronosticari circa superfluitatem secunde digestionis, scilicet circa urinam pariter cum ydropisi. Quare laudat bonam urinam per bonam ypostasim, profert (134rB) diffinitionem continentis ex contento. Ex hoc dicit Ysaac actio nature membrorum prefixum et determinatum habet terminum, ut suam actionem perficiat neque alterius perficere valeat. Ex hoc enim intelligitur quod unum membrum non complet inperfectionem alterius. Si tertia digestio est bona, et secunda et

---

[87] *fortasse* humoribus *vice* habentibus
[88] *fortasse* longae *vice* longi

prima precessit bona. Si prima digestio est mala, et secunda et tertia erit mala, ad quod notandum quod natura summa et provida quedam membra instituit in quibus cibus captaretur et habilior efficeretur ad inmutationem instituit os et stomachum. Ore enim cibus commasticatur, non de facili immutetur[89] ad digestionem. Hoc modo stomachum ordinavit ut esset albi coloris ut in actione esset subtilis substantie et frigide et sicce nature. Cibus veniens ad stomachum immutatur a stomacho cuiuscumque coloris si fit alibi[90] coloris subtilis substantie quam preparatus erat exire, unde per frigiditatem eiusdem et siccitatem has qualitates habentes motum ad centrum retinetur ne exeat. Si consideremus alia membra nullum inveniemus eiusdem nature ut si mala digestio sit in stomacho non potest[91] suppleri in alio membro. Epar membrum est calidum et humidum purpurei coloris. Purpureus color compositus est ex rubeo at nigro et utcumque albo et est terrestris substantie. Nullum membrum in corpore ab ispo hoc habet, unde si mala celebratur digestio in epate mala erit in omnibus membris. In fontibus enim terminatur actio digestionis, digestio enim cum sit actio nature in fontibus terminatur, quelibet enim actio nature tripplici clauditur termino, primo medio et fine; et cuius finis bonus est ipsum quoque bonum est, unde si bona tertia digestio, bona prima et secunda; si bona tertia digestio, bona est eius superfluitas; si bona superfluitas bonus sanguis, si bonus sanguis bona eius materia; si bona materia, bona actio per quam fuit generatus; sed generatus fuit per secundam digestionem, ergo bona secunda digestio et sic bona eius superfluitas, ergo si bona urina bona ypostasis. In ypostasi tria attenduntur principaliter, quartum hiis tribus dicitur adiacere. (134vA) Principaliter attenditur color albus, positio in fundo, et continuitas substantie cum forma pineata. Quartum hiis tribus adiacet: hoc est, equalitas temporis iuxta illud, hoc est equale in tempore. In tempore servato albus color laudatur et ypostasis significat per effectionem motus alterativi qui exigitur ad opus tercie digestionis, necesse namque fuit alteranda a propria forma expoliari sanguis namque rubore perfusus alterationem suscipiens. Tum ex immutatione membrorum, tum ex calore excoquente, propria forma expoliatur et sumit aqueam formam et ne dum sanguis immo eius superfluitas, scilicet ypostasis, sicut enim aqua elementum nulll medio transit in terram, sic necesse fuit sanguinem esse album quod paratur transire in terrestrem membrorum essentiam. Continuitas substantie declarat perfectionem motus localis facti in tertia digestione. Necesse fuit partium fieri transpositionem partibus in sua positione malum et cetera, non enim in alteratione sanguinis virtus peccavit, quia consumpta est per calorem. Fumositas impellens vel

divellens forme fuit pineate ex fortitudine caloris, naturalis calor namque motum habet de centro, ispum consequendo circa rem aliam incipit a diffusione latitudinis et elongando protenditur in acutum quod videtur in flamma, cui naturaliter inest caliditas, quia ipsa incipit a diffusione latitudinis et cetera. Hoc secundum grecos sortitur ignis ut dicatur "pir," id est, charbons acutum,[92] cum inferiori diffusione latitudinis, inde piramides, sepulcra antiquorum. Caliditas igitur terrestria ipsius sediminis immixta aquosis cum diffusione in inferiori parte locavit, aërea tanquam subtilia super ea, ignea tanquam acuta suprema; positio in fundo declarat perfectionem motus essentialis. Necesse fuit substantie et forme in aliud esse fieri transitum. Membra terrestria sanguinem in terrestritatem commutant et ne dum sanguis suscipit terrestritatem, immo eius superfluitas, quare ex parcium terrestritate fundum petit. Equalitas temporis exigitur ut per (134vB) severet cum illis differentiis ex quo apparet usque ad creticam determinationem perseverantium[93] differentiarum, perfectio enim motuum tertie digestionis et virtutis immutative secunde. *Urina bo[na] est que habet ypostasim albam:* talis urina merito bona est quia est cum proprio colore et propria substantia tum quia perficit celebrata est. Est tertia digestio in membris et si bona est tertia digestio, bona fuit prima et secunda. Est cum proprio colore, scilicet cum rufo, qui significat tenperantiam qualitatum passivarum. Quare albus color laudatur in ypostasi et vituperatur in natura? Alibi solvitur, et *subsi[dentem]*, id est, in fundo existentem partium terrestritatem. Terrestria tanquam gravia de sui natura fundum petunt; *et equalem* ut equalis sit perseverantia ut sicut hodie apparuerit ita et cras appareat. Vel ut dicunt alii *equalem precedenti vel subsequenti et continuam*, propter ventositatis defectum, et *levem*, non scrupulosam, *et personalis*, ut sit simplex relatio et non personalis, quia urina que nigra in primo non perseveret usque ad crisim. Et *permansit usque in crisim*, id est, sit perseverantia huius bonitatis in qualicumque urina, *usque ad crisim*, id est, usque ad morbi declinationem, talis determinatio fit ad bonum quia fit ex vigore nature. *Est enim u[na nuncia] fi[delis] spe[rande] sa[lutis]*: pro vigore virtutum naturalium et perfectione digestionum. Vigor virtutum naturalium et perfectio digestionum indicant fortitudinem caloris naturalis, calor enim naturalis virtutes vivificat. Natura namque consimilium pariter est inmutata natura offitii et utrorumque unde spes est de futura salute. *Quod si modo cum ypostasi p[redicta] mo[do] si[ne] e[a] fu[erit] di[uturnitatem] egri[tudinis] si[gnificat]*: et nature debilitatem que aliquando movetur ad superflua expellenda aliquando non, debilis, aut natura debilis deficit dum vires morbi prevalent et ideo quandoque debilitata succumbit, nec omnino fidelis quia in dubium ponit medicum.

---

[89] *fortasse* immutatur *vice* immutetur
[90] *fortasse* sit albi *vice* fit alibi
[91] *fortasse* possit *vice* potest

[92] *fortasse* charbon accensum *vice* charbons acutum
[93] perseverantium *legitur vice* perseverantiam *in codice*

25. *Urina rubea ni[mis]*: auctor superius ostendit bonam urinam cum bona ypostasi brevitatem declarare egritudinis, nunc intendit ostendere minus bonam urinam cum ypostasi sibi declarare simili egritudinem diuturnam. (135rA) Rubor in urina multum existens et ypostasi significat multitudinem sanguinis tingentis substantiam urine et ypostasis. Ex sanguinis ergo multitudine prolixa est egritudo, multa enim materia non potest brevi tempore digeri. Sed tamen quia sanguis est humor digestibilis et amicus humane nature significatur ad bonum egritudo determinetur.[94] *Urina ru[bea] ni[mis]*, id est, rubicunda; *cum sibi simili ypostasi*, id est, rubicunda vel subrubicunda, *diu[turnitatem] egri[tudinis] magis su[perioribus] dicit:* pro multitudine sanguinis peccantis quantitative, multus sanguis diuturnam significat egritudinem. *Est tamen nun[cia] cer[ta] et fi[delis] sperande sa[lutis]*: non declarat humorem furiosum esse in calore neque crudum sed sanguineum que calidus est et humidus habens qualitates vivificatorias et per suas qualitates iuvat digestionem et se iuvat digeri et membris in corpora. Et *si eiusdem ypostasis fur[furea]*: ypostasis furfurea aut est alba aut rubea aut[95] liquefactionem membrorum demonstrat et resolutionem, rubea sanguinis adustionem, sanguis adustus, quia minus habilis est ad digerendum, prolixiorem indicat egritudinem. Furfurea ypostasis existens rubea mala est, quia secundum speciem ethice insinuat que incurabilis est. Iam calor membris est insertus consumens humiditatem corporis in longum et latum. Pessima est squamosa, quia maiorem significat dissolutionem. Squamose resolutiones in urina fiunt a vescica quia vescica alba est et concava; similiter squame concave et alba; et si calor fortis potuit dissolvere vescicam in squamas, membrum frigidum et durum et expositum, quid facit in intrinsecis ubi proprie et magis [calor] viget quid in membris calidis mollibus tota eorum exausta est humiditas. Alba autem et liquida licet ypostasis sit, superfluitas tercie digestionis. Hic per hypostasim intelligamus humores flegmaticos in inferiori urine regione apparentes quia res gravis de natura sui petit inferiora. Si humores flegmatici appareant in urina indicant materiam frigidam, longum tempus expos(135rB)tulat ad sui digestionem. *Alba ergo ypostasis*, propter immutationem flegmaticorum humorum, *et liquida*, id est, clara, *mala est:* quia materia ultra modum est cruda; *peior tamen que dicta est furfurea:* quia firmiores partes significat resolvi.

26. *Nebula pendens in urina et cetera:* notandum est quod sedimen tercie digestionis secundum tripplicem locum tria sumit vocabula. Apparens in fundo dicitur ypostasis ab "ypos," quod est "sub," et "stasis," "stans," eo quod subtus eius est stare; apparens in medio dicitur "emorroyda," hoc est, "dependens"; apparens in superficie dicitur "nephilis,"

vel "nubes," id est, ad similitudinem nubium. Notandum quod quodlibet horum sediminum potest dici nebula, id est, corpus nebulosum quia substantia urine obnubilat. Ypostasis alba significat summum bonum, encorrima album minus bonum, nephilis alba longe minus bonum. Ypostasis nigra declarat summum malum, encorrima nigrum minus malum, nephilis nigra longe minus malum. Ypostasis [alba] significat summum bonum, significat perfectionem tercie digestionis per quam sanguis dealbatus est, et est prout debet esse merito. Si superfluitas sanguinis fuit eiusdem coloris prout sanguis, significat summum bonum. Minus bonum significat encorrima album, ex eo enim quod pendet, et est substantia encorrimatis; elevata mala est, significatur ventositatis presentia generante[96] ex debilitate caloris naturalis, non enim calor fuit fortis qui debuit consumere ventositatem. Nephilis alba longe minus malum significat quia maiorem copiam ventositatis significat potentis cordis sediminis[97] ad superiora elevare, et quanto maior est copia ventositatis, tanto maior est debilitas caloris naturalis. Ypostasis nigra significat summum malum quia adustionem vel mortificationem significat in terrestri substantia. Precedente colore viridi significat adustionem, precedenti livido significat mortificationem. Minus malum encorrima nigrum quia minus terrestris est substantie, tam encorrima quam ypostasis (135vA), unde minorem significat mortificationem vel adustionem. Nephilis nigra pro subtilitate substantie significat principium adustionis vel mortificationis, unde lo[n]ge minus malum significat. *Nebula pendens in urina:* hic nebula largo modo accipitur pro ypostasi quia corpus est nebulosum; *pendens*, id est, apparens. *Si alba bona:* quia summum declarat bonum; *nigra mala*, quia summum malum. *Dum urina citri[na] et cla[ra] fu[erit] indi[gesta] egri[tudinis prolixitatem] significat:* scilicet materiam indigestam. Notandum quod licet urina non tingatur a calore extraneo sed a naturali, secundum quod dicit Constantinus calor extraneus operatur in ipsius urine colorationem preparando materiam ineptam ipsam, dissolvendo et rarefaciendo, unde si calor non debilis sit naturalis inveniens materiam preparatam consequitur in ea quod suum est [et] eius partes igneas multiplicat. Videmus enim quod aliquis cultello carnes crudas incidendo[98] efficiuntur habiles ad coquendum, unde debilis calor poterit eas excoquere. Urina citrina in egritudine et perseverans significat debilitatem caloris naturalis, qui non potest immutare ipsam et si calor in principio et in augmento quando utcumque fortis fuit non potuit immutare, minus immutabit quando debilior erit, unde prolixitate caloris processu temporis patiens succumberet, et talis urina si fuerit per siccitatem siccitas inferendo partes humores

94 *fortasse* determinatur *vice* determinetur
95 *fortasse* rubea alba *vice* rubea aut
96 *fortasse* generate *vice* generante
97 cordis sediminis divellente *Vat 43rA*
98 *fortasse legitur* quando aliquis . . . incidit

compactiores efficiuntur unde perseverat indigestio, *unde ti[mendus] est infir[mi] de[fectus]:* propter prolixitatem egritudinis qua natura debilitatur. *Urina [aquosa] significativa mortis:* sed per aquosam urinam denotatur alba, quia aquosa dicitur ab aqua. Urina alba veniens in principio est fidelis, id est, certa nuncia mortis quia significat prolixitatem egritudinis et ex eo ipsi[99] infirmi defectum, in fine vero si veniat pauca et malis signis perseverantibus, mala est, ut in frenesi, quia significat materiam retineri et extinctionem significat naturalis caloris. Si eveniat multa in fine, bonis signis perseverantibus, bona, quia significat materiam solvi et purgari. *Fetens mala est:* inbeccillitatem significat caloris naturalis non valentis depu(135vB)rare subiectum a superfluis, quia quod caliditas dissolvit calor naturalis consumit. Superflua aggregata et non depurata malum dant odorem que immutat urinam unde urina fetida est. Fetidus odor significat corruptionem humorum agentium ad corruptionem, *fidelis dicitur,* id est, fidelem dans [nuntium] mortis; *nigra* mala est, quia significat adustionem vel mortificationem; *lutuosa*[100] *ma[la] est,* quia solidorum humorum significat habundantiam perturbantium urinam. In utroque sexu nimis pessimam, quasi diceret non solum in viris est pessima sed in viris et mulieribus. Magis ex precedenti viridi pessima est in viris propter adustionem, nigra ex precedenti livido pessima est in mulieribus propter mortificationem. *In pueris vero aquosa urina ma[la] est:* dicunt quidam quia natura puerorum est caliditas et humiditas, declarat talis urina permutationem duarum qualitatum deputatarum in tali etate, scilicet, caliditatis et humiditatis, *vel quod natura aquosa,* id est, unctuosa, mala est in pueris propter substantiam[101] labilem significat puerum liquari. *Urina clara,* id est, tenuis et *cruda,* id est, alba et *diuturna,* diu apparens cum aliis signis bona cum facili actione inspirandi et respirandi, *certum est apostema futurum sub diafragma[te],* id est, in nutritivis, albus color fit per frigiditatem multiplicantem aquosas partes et aquosos humores, unde alba urina significat frigidorum humorum habundantiam. Ex eo enim quod tenuis est siccitatem significat agentem ad compactionem humorum unde est egritudinem prolixari et egrum debilitari. Virtus debilis nequid perfectam celebrare crisim, et quia materia gravis est quod perpenditur propter frigiditatem et compactionem ipsius habet inferius determinari et non superius, unde est quod pocius colligitur sub diafragmate quam superius. *Cras[sicies] ut ara[nee] te[la] superna[tans] urine vitu[peranda] est:* significat enim resolutionem pinguedinis, unde auctor addit *significat egrum liquari,* id est, liquefieri. *Rationis est et ordinem et in ne[bula] non ne[gligere]:* triplex namque positio attendenda est in sedimine, inferior, media

et superior. (136rA) Antepositum sedimen potest nebula appellari quia sui interpositione nebulosum reddit corpus urine, hic ostenditur nebula pro ypostasi, appellatio ypostasis namque. *An tenet medium locum aut supremum,* id est, aut est in medio calicis aut inferius, et *col[orem] similiter,* cum albo in medio albi coloris existens significat minus bonum, superius longe minus bonum. *Que enim est media cum predicto co[lore],* id est, cum albo; *lau[dabilis] est,* id est, minus mala quam alba nephilis, *supprema vero nigra vituperabilis,* id est, inferior vituperabilis est per terrestrium membrorum adustionem. *Ca[vendum] est [ne]*[102] *vitio vesice ca[piaris]:* aliquando furfurea ypostasis provenit a vescica quandoque a toto corpore. Docet auctor quandoque provenit a vescica, quando a toto corpore: furfurea facta, a vescica cum spissa substantia furfurea, a toto corpore cum tenui substantia. *Medicus vero ergo caveat:* sibi ne capiatur vitio vescice, quia forte vitium est in vescica et tale vitium dicit a toto corpore provenire. *Vel quod est eius vitium dic[it] alie[num] indicat:* quod si alterius et ista levior: est littera.

27. [*Prognostics* XIII] *Vomitus lau[dabilis] et cetera:* auctor intendit pronosticari circa vomitum, id est, circa id quod per vomitum educitur, quia multipliciter consideratur in quantitate, qualitate et tempore. In quantitate quia aut multus aut paucus et tam multus quam paucus aut fit vi nature aut fit vi sinthomatis. Multus vi nature quando nociva materia prehendat in superiori regione nutritivorum, unde tota a corpore per vomitum educitur, et ex tali eductione eger levior et suavior efficitur; paucus fit vi nature, quando natura per aliam regionem fere expulit quam superiorem regionem, unde parum remanet in superiori regione unde paucus vomitus. Multus vi sinthomatis vel fit ex qualitate materiei aut furiositate eiusdem, vel fit ex multitudine quando multa est et viscosa, vel ex membrorum incontinentia ut fit[103] materiosa: quando cibaria sicut mittuntur eiciuntur. Paucus vi sinthomatis quando furiosa est materia (136rB) et subtile quod est de ea educitur quod petit superiora, unde paucus vomitus. In qualitate consideratur in colore, odore, sapore, tenuitate et spissitudine. In colore considerari debet subcitrinus, subcitrinus color laudatur, qui declarat temperantiam duarum qualitatum activarum, scilicet caliditatis et frigiditatis, moderantiam duorum humorum naturaliter immissorum ad stomachum, scilicet flegmatis et colere. Iterum [si] fuerit citrinus declarat habundantiam colere et cetera. In odore consideratur si fuerit fetidi odoris profundam declarat corruptionem humorum, si fuerit gravis principium corruptionis membrorum declarat. In sapore consideratur, nam si fuerit acetosi saporis vel melancoliam vel flegma acetosum et cetera. In tenuitate et spissitudine, si fuerit subtilis et tenuis si[c] subtilium et fluidorum

---

[99] *fortasse* ipsius *vice* ipsi
[100] *fortasse* lutosa *vice* lutuosa
[101] *fortasse* substantialem *vice* substantiam

[102] vi *reduplicatur vice* ne *in codice*
[103] *fortasse* sit *vice* fit

humorum declarat habundantiam, [si] spisse crossorum humorum; in tempore ut fiat in die cretico. Dicit auctor: *Lau[dabilis] vo[mitus] cui flegma admixtum co[lere] fuerit*, id est, qui provenit ex admixtione colere et flegmatis, colera enim non excedit ut inducat croceum colorem neque flegma album, sed ex alterutra contradictione subcitrinus provenit color. *Neque nimis viscosus:* neque mediocris substantie debet esse ut declaret temperantiam qualitatum passivarum, non prevalet siccitas rarefaciens ut si sit subtilis non humiditas ut sit spisse substantie. *Quanto vero ab hac sim[plicitate] re[motior]:* a simplici natura, non habens in se malitiam sicut dicitur homo simplex, *vel ab hac simplici[tate] remotior*, id est, ab hac singulari et propria bonitate tanto suspectior, quia non declarat temperantiam neque moderantiam. *Vomitus ut sucus porrorum:* qui declarat principium adustionis; *vel viridis*, maiorem adustionem; *aut plumbeus*, principium mortificationis; *aut niger* vel mortificationem vel adustionem. *Ma[lum] est si omnibus hiis infectum fu[erit] coloribus:* quia diversi humores in stomacho prehendant ut colera eruginosa, vel ex diversa actione qualitatum exuberantium diver(136vA)si proveniunt colores, nedum cum omnes predicti colores apparentes declarant pernitiem, immo unius mortis nuntius est. *Continuus omnis dolor malus:* sive fuerit gravis odor sive fetidus in quocumque vomitu declarante malitia[m] malum est.

28. [*Prognostics* XIIII] *Sputum in omni acuta egri[tudine] et cetera:* auctor intendit pronosticari circa sputum. Sputum a tribus membris educitur, scilicet, a cerebro, stomacho et pulmone. Veniens a cerebro exit cum rascatione, a pulmone cum excreatione educitur vel tussicula, a stomacho simpliciter educitur. Sputum enim licet ab hiis tribus membris educatur, proprie a pulmone educitur. Est autem flegmatica superfluitas in pulmone generata, iuxta illud quod frigidum est et humidum in secunda digestione, hoc trahit ad se pulmo ad flegmatis generationem. Sputum igitur egritudinum ibi vel circa illum locum contingentium est declarativum, ut pleuresis et peripleumonie. Pleuresis est apostema factum in teneritatibus costarum; peripleumonia est apostema factum iuxta pulmonem, scilicet, in pulmonis casula, et dicitur peripleumonia a pery, quod est "circum," et "plegmio," id est, "pulmo," eo quod fiat iuxta pulmonem et non in ipsa pulmonis substantia ut quidam opinantur. Sputum multipliciter consideratur, in quantitate, qualitate, tempore et modo exitus. In quantitate sputum consideratur quia aliud multum aliud paucum et tam paucum quam multam aut fit vi nature aut vi sinthomatis. Multum factum vi nature quoniam nocivam materiam bene digestam a corpore educit; ex tali eductione eger levior et suavior efficitur vel in salutem restituitur. Paucus fit vi nature quando nocivam materiam fere

ex toto per poros venarum subintrat, venatis[104] ad epar transducit et ab epate ad quilim et a quili ad renes et cum urina emittitur. Multum fit vi sinthomatis vel ex quantitate vel ex membrorum incontinentia. Paucum vi sinthomatis fit vel ex mortificatione vel adjustione vel ex defectu virtutis expulsive In qualitate multipliciter consideratur, in colore, odore, sapore, tenuitate et spissitudine. (136vB) In colore, debet enim esse subrubeum, sano sputo admixtum, a septimo die incipiat apparere aliter. Subrubeum enim laudatur quia declarat materiam sanguineam, utraque qualitate obediente digestioni in coenum quod est sano sputo admixtum declaratur quod corpus non multum sit permutatum a priori consistentia. In eo enim quod a septimo die apparet aliud declarat fortitudinem naturalis caloris circa locum excoctionis nocive materiei cum fortitudine virtutis digestive. Item si fuerit rubei coloris declarat habundantiam sanguinis et cetera. In odore consideratur, quia fetidum pernitiosum est, quia declarat corruptionem humorum gravi membrorum corruptione. In sapore ut dictum est in sudore. In tempore quia debet fieri in die cretico, in modo exitus quia aut fit cum angustia aut sine angustia. Dicit auctor: *Sputum in omni egritudine pul[monis]:* scilicet peripleumonia, *seu coste*, ut in pleuresi, *utile est [si] velox:* propter fortitudinem virtutis expulsive, seu facile propter obedientiam materiei ad digestionem. *Si sine la[bore]:* per quod removetur cruditas, viscositas, adustio, cumulatio in unum non circumdat, ut urina laboret neque viscosa, *si subrubeum*, quod significat materiam sanguineam conscentientem digestioni et sano sputo commixto, quia corpus non est permutatum a priori. *Si vero tardium[105]* ad eductionem vi[scositatis] natura laborat pro viscositate vel cruditate vel adustione vel cumulatione, *in do[loris] principio*, ed est, in confirmatione apostematis dolorem praestante, *pessimum est*, quod declarat materiam furiosam et *rubeum* pro venarum excoriatione ex materia furiosa proveniente, *aut ci[trinum]*, quod declarat coleram esse in caliditate. *Cum labo[riosa] tussi:* quod videtur tussire et nil expellit pro viscositate materiei retinetur humor. *Neque sano sputo admistum:* per quod declarat quod corpus permutatum sit a priori consistentia. *Rubeum omnino mo[lestum]:* quia [de]clarat rupturam venarum in pulmone, *album*, quod declarat indigestionem, *viscosum*, per siccitatem inserentem, *globosum*, per frigiditatem mortificantem, *viride spu[mosum]*, quod declarat adustionem *malum, et si ni[grum] pes[simum]:* (137rA) quia mortificatione; et *si in pul[mone] so[nuerit]:* propter frigiditatem mortificantem vel siccitatem inserentem *nequicquam exi[erit] malum*, unde declaratur vigor siccitatis inserentis quando fit malus sonus in fine vite qui dicitur oresinon.

---

[104] *fortasse* venulis *vice* venatis
[105] *fortasse* tardum *sive* tardivum *vice* tardium

29. *Sternutatio cum reumate:* pronosticatur auctor circa sternutationem.   Sternutatio est sonus violente commotionis cerebri vel violenta cerebri commotio in fortitudine virtutis expulsive et debilitate virtutis retentive persistens, cum cerebrum movetur ad superflua expellenda quibus opprimitur.   *Sternutatio cum re[umate]*, id est, cum humoris fluxu reumatico; reuma est fluxus humorum ad aliquam partem corporis, et hic fluxus humorum reumaticus fit ad spiritualia ubi colligitur materia ad apostema peripleumonicum.   Omnis dolor exacuit reuma et ad locum dolentem confluunt humores.   *Sternu[tatio] cum reu[mate]*: ubi adest confluxus violentus reumatizans, *in omni egri[tudine] pul[monis] et coste*, ut in pleuresi et peripleumonia, *malum est;* materia apostematis replet et per humorem fluentem fit maior dolor et maior fluxus, unde maior repletio et fit suffocatio. *Sive enim stern[ut]atio precedat*, cum fluxu violento, *sive co[equa] sit*, id est, comitetur, *malum est*, propter violentiam humoris reumatizantis et fluentis et collectionem ad apostema ducentis.   *Sternu[tatio] in omni egritudine sine re[umate]*, sine violento fluxu humoris, bonum est; cerebrum existens forte expellit humorem qui potest colligi ad apostema, unde fit sternutatio.   Sputum subsanguineum: quedam premiserat auctor de sputato, iam de eo subiungit. *Spu[tum] subsan[guineum] clarum:* non habens perturbationem humorum per quod declaratur quod sit sano sputo admixtum, unde fortitudo infirmi morbum suum tolerare potentis per hoc declaratur. *In pul[monis] vali[tudine] in principio salutem significat:* quia declaratur quod materia obediens utraque qualitati digestioni obediens, *si usque in septimum diem aut amplius* (137rB) *idem sputum*, id est, eadem maneries sputi *manserit suspectum est:* quia si in principio egritudinis non potuit digere[re] materiam utraque qualitate conscentientem digestioni in augmento quando erit debilis minus operabitur. *Omne spu[tum] perse[verante] do[lore] ma[lum] est:* quia materia est furiosa vel multa, unde furiositate dissipat unde multitudinem replet et suffocat spiritualia.[106]   *Omnis do[lor] pre[dictorum] locorum*, ut in pulmone vel costis, *superve[niente] spu[to] vel solutione ventris; fit solutio* ventris quando fit collectio ad apostema in diafragmate et ut dicit Ysaac in Viatico fit pleuresis non vera.   Materia illa venatis[107] mittitur ad stomachum et recipitur in concavitate stomachi et inducit ventris solutionem. *Vel flebotomo adhabito[108] vel quolibet compe[tenti] medicamine*, dando diuretica, et *do[lor] non fu[erit] di[minutus] pus ibi denunciat futurum:* quia materia illa concludatur[109] et in pus convertitur. *Pu[tredo] colerica:* dixerat auctor superius [quod] omnis dolor

predictorum locorum superveniente sputo vel solutione ventris vel flebotomo adhabito ˙ [dolor] non fuerit diminutus pus ibi denunciat.   Ne ergo aliquis putaret quod quelibet determinatio putredinis fieret ad bonum remover auctor per presentem litteram dicens, *pu[tredo] co[lerica]*, que viridis est vel nigra sputo commixta sano.   Intelligas quod sputum si per se apparet et non cum putredine colerica sanitatis esset declarativum.   *Malum est:* malum enim declarat putredo cum sit viridis vel nigra, adustionem declarat [et] furiosam se indicat unde sui furiositate dissecando membra dissipat et corrumpit.   Et *maxime si a die septimo con[tingat]:* quasi diceret si in principio apparet putredo colerica non est ita suspecta ut a septimo die in antea, quia calor naturalis existens in principio vigorosus circa materiam illam diutius in saniem transducit, et si a septimo die in antea apparet calor naturalis non fuerit fortis in principio ut transduceret materiam in saniem.   Tunc enim transduxit in saniem, quando valde debilitatur et si debilitatur calor naturalis qui regitivus est corporis humani (137vA) debilitantur virtutes unde machina humani corporis pacienti est sarcina. *Mortem namque in quartodecimo die pronunciabis:* quia augmentum egritudinis ubi apparet talis putredo colerica differtur usque ad undecimum diem unde materia per tantum spatium debilitatur unde mortem iudicabis in quartodecimo die, quia materia magis est furiosa et natura magis debilis.   Et non simpliciter mortem debemus predicere, *nisi signum sperandum[110] salutis adesse consideraveris quod huiusmodi est*, id est, nisi maneries signorum declarantium salutem apparuerit; *quod huiusmodi est huius maneries robur et constantis egri:* per quod declaratur fortitudo caloris naturalis, ergo abscentia cruditatis removetur in materia namque fortitudo caloris naturalis opposita est cruditati materiei et tenperata habundantia humorum declaratur que contraria est furiositati materiei: *bo[nus] spiritus*, id est, bona actio inspirandi et respirandi propter defectum aduste materiei suffocantis, et non impedientis actionem inspirandi et respirandi non adest multitudo materiei operans ad suffocationem cum sit suffocatio spiritus offenditur; et *facilis proiectio putredinis cum tussi:* quia fortis est virtus expulsiva que non laborat in proiciendo, non est impedita ab humore vel humoribus ab aliqua qualitate vel qualitatibus contrariis; *et equalitas tocius corporis in habitu[dine]* caloris, scilicet, secundum dispositionem caloris quia calor equaliter disponit interiora et exteriora, exposita membra et non exposita, nobilia et ignobilia, per quod removetur suspictio apostematis non intus innati, pro quo interiora dolentia traheretur spiritus ad interiora et exteriora frigerent; et *mollitu[do] ca[loris][111]* aut moderatus aut immoderatus: immoderatus dissolvit et consumit unde prestat duritiem; moderatus dissolvendo tantum et consumendo pre-

---

[106] *Post* spiritualia *additur:* Omne sputum cum doloris dimintione bonum est *Vat 44rV*
[107] *cf.* note 104 *supra*
[108] adhibito *Vat 44rB*
[109] *fortasse* concludetur *vice* concludatur

---

[110] *nisi signum sperande Vat 44rB*
[111] mollitudinis vice mollitudo caloris *Vat 44rB*

stat mollitiem et ex hoc adest defectus accidentalis caloris. *Neque sitierit:* quia non deficit nutrimentum (137vB) quod declarat bonam dispositionem epatis et membrorum nutrientium fortem virtutem; et *stercus,* quod declarat bonam virtutem [et bonam] dispositionem stomachi et intestinorum, et *sudor* qui declarat bonam dispositionem tocius corporis, et *sompnus* qui declarat bonam dispositionem animatorum membrorum, *bene se habuerit,* id est, non existentia quomodolibet impedita, *vitam sunt polli[centia],* id est, signa pronostica future vite eliciuntur. *Ex quibus si de[fuerint] plura mā[lum],* id est, si aliquorum signorum fuerit defectus quia bona pauciora sunt quam debet esse *mor[tem] fu[turam] confir[mabis]:* deficiunt bona et emergunt plura mala et quare mors supervenit propter nature debilitatem. Notandum est hic quod sit[112] tot sint bona quot mala, et efficatoria[113] bona quam mala indica[nt] salutem; si efficatoria mala, mortem. Et *contrarium quod est mors,* id est, alia sunt signa mortis per contrarium supradicta per quod mors elicitur. *Huiusmodi est id est sic attenduntur debi[litas] egri anxius spiritus magnus et densus perma[nens] proiectio cum laboriosa tussi:* pro debilitate virtutis expulsive sitis [adest] per se, propter succensionem colerice materiei spiritualia distemperantur in calore, calidum[114] fumositates dessiccant os stomachi, vel sitis adest propter defectum nutrimenti. *[Circa] corporis [caloris] inequalitas:* pro presentia apostematis nati interius, unde membra frigescunt extrinseca compacientia in interioribus unde frigescunt ventris; et *la[terum] ca[lor] magnus,* propter calidas fumositates et calefacientes sed frontis et manuum et pedum frigor quia calor extinguitur illas partes primo derelinquit quas ultro expetit; et *urina* que declarat malam dispositionem stomachi, et *sudor* qui declarat inperfectionem digestionis et malam dispositionem tocius corporis, et *sompnus* qui insinuat malam dispositionem membrorum animatorum. Hec omnia ut diximus sunt minantia *mortem fu[turam],* id est, proximam; *hec signa si predicte proiectioni[s] colerice materie super[venerint]:* ipsa sufficit ad pernitionem. *Mor[tem] fu[turam] ante quattuordecimum die[m] non du[bitabis]* (138rA) nedum ista *aut in nono,* natura existente valde debili, *aut in undecimo,* natura existente utcumque debili. *In hac con[sideratione] spu[tum] dices esse mor[tale],* id est, propter predictam considerationem, et *si vitalia,* id est, signa declarantia vitam rationabiliter investiges, *vel mortis signa co[gnoveris] pro[nosticorum] recti[tudine] inoffen[se] progredieris,* quia victurum ascribes vite, moriturum morti.

30. *Apostematum et cetera:* varias determinationes apostematum in subsequentibus auctor posuerat et prefixum terminum rupture earum terminationum

non insinuerat. Ideo prefixit determinationis rupture apostematis assignare intendit, quia apostematum aliud colericum aliud sanguineum aliud flegmaticum aliud melancolicum. Sanguinem apostema differt sui rupturam infra vicesimum diem que[115] habet duas qualitates plurimum concordantes corruptioni, materialem scilicet humiditatem et artificialem scilicet caliditatem. Apostema flegmaticum differt rupturam sui in vicesimo die, quia licit habeat frigiditatem discrepantem corruptioni habet humiditatem que potissima est et concordantem corruptioni. Apostema colericum differt rupturam sui in quadragesimo [die] licet habeat causam artificialem, scilicet caliditatem habet tamen siccitatem nimium dissentientem corruptioni. Apostema melancolicum differt rupturam sui in quinquagesimo [die] quia utraque sui qualitate discrepat que cita[116] non fit corruptio et hoc est quod dicit. *Apostematum quedam in vicesimo,* ut apostema sanguineum infra diem vicesimum et apostema flegmaticum in vicesimo, *quedam in quadragesimo,* ut apostema colericum, *quedam in sexagesimo,* ut apostema melancolicum, *rupturam differt. Oportet me[dicum] diem principii non ignorare:* medicus nature minister non ygnarus debet attendere diem principii multiplici ex causa ut videat motus egritudinis, aut per rupturam ternariam aut per quaternariam, et visis signis digestionis materiei propinet farmatiam in die (138rB) cretico. Sed natura ad diversa non valet esse attenta, littera sic continuatur, quia varia sunt genera apostematum et in diversis temporibus fiunt eorum determinationes ex quibus et in quibus medicus posset decipi. *Oportet ergo medicum diem principii non igno[rare]:* principium aliud est ante [feb]rem, aliud cum [feb]re, aliud tempus egritudinis; principium ante [feb]rem quando solummodo sola causa antecedens egri est in corpore; principium cum [feb]re est motus egritudinis quando corpus incipit calere aut primo frigere preter naturam; principium tempus egritudinis quando egritudo differt usque ad quartum diem, quando durat in undecimo die, quandoque in sextodecimo die, et secundum Galenum usque ad centesimum et hoc est quod dicit. *Oportet medicum diem principii non igno[rare]:* diem principii, non tempus egritudinis, non principii ante [feb]rem, sed principii cum [feb]re. *In qua hora corpus primo habuerit calorem aut fri[gidi-tatem][117] preter naturam quando ceperit in eo lo[co] [dolere] et compunctio[nes] senti[re]:* pro discursu humoris ad apostema colligendum, et etiam medicus non ignorare debet maneriem doloris utrum dolor ille sit infixivus, pungitivus, aggravatus vel extensivus. Nam si fuerit infixivus dices determinationes fieri infra vicesimum, si extensivus in vicesimo, si pungitivus in quadragesimo, si aggravatus in sexagesimo. *Hec enim sunt prima collectionis inditia:*

---

[112] *fortasse* si *vice* sit
[113] *fortasse* efficatiora *vice* efficatoria
[114] *fortasse* calidae *vice* calidum

[115] *fortasse* quia *vice* que
[116] *fortasse* cito *vice* cita
[117] In quo corpus primo habuerit calere aut frigere *Vat 44vB*

scilicet, calefactio vel infrigidatio; natura nam dum materia colligitur ad apostema incipit dolor qualis solvitur continuitas; omnis dolor exacuit reuma, spiritus distemperantur in calore et sic calet corpus preter naturam. *Ex quo*, id est, tempore collectionis, *computanda erit tibi dies hinc quoque eruptionem in predicta tempora exspec[tabis]*: aut in vicesimo aut in quadragesimo aut sexagesimo et *si col[lectio] in uno laterum*[118] *conti[gerit] ad apostema*, faciendum aut in ambobus. Videndum est utrum sit in uno laterum vel in ambobus, *si in uno la[terum] utiliter percunc[taberis]*, perquires et quomodo perquiremus; *si in altero*, id est, supero, *magis caluerit*, dicemus ibi fieri collectionem et quia in altero latere non est apostema. *Iubebis iacere super alterum*: (138vA) ut quiescat locus ubi fit collectio, et *si in altero*, ubi iacet, *pondus sederit*, pro discursu humoris ad apostema. Et si non senserit *ex hoc*, id est, ex hac consideratione, *tamen dices apostema in uno la[terum] et non in ambobus*. Et alia sunt collectionum inditia, *ex signis huius[modi] que sunt putribilia*, quasi diceret alia collectionum inditia per hec signa dignoscitur: *fe[bris] erit in[deficiens]*, quia dum spiritus mittuntur ad locum dolentem, distemperantur in calore et propter continuam transmissionem et distemperantiam, febris adest indeficiens; sed *in die mo[dica]*, propter hoc quia anima vacat ab intrinsecis operationibus perficiendis unde spiritus non ita distemperantur, neque humores *in nocte magis accensa*: quia reumatica causa magis movetur de nocte quam de die unde maior transmissio spirituum et sic maior distemperantia; *sudor multus et in tussiendo falsa quies*: propter apostema spiritualium opprimitur tracea arteria, et fit offendiculum, et fit tussis. Falsa quies est, videntur quiescere modicum et statim tussire videntur, et *oculorum reductio* ad exteriora, propter fumositates impellentes oculorum que dum transmittuntur ad oculos que habeant collimitantiam cum spiritualibus, *atque in eorum angulis rubor*, propter pu[n]cturam fumositatum facientium apertionem venarum unde sanguis exit et rubeum prestat colorem, *et unguium constrictio*, propter caliditatem et siccitatem quia siccitatis est constringere, *et digitorum calor*, propter calidas fumositates transmissas ad digitos. *Amplius tamen in eorundem summi[tati]bus*: quia calor habet motum de centro, magis potens est in exterioribus; *et in pe[di]bus fiunt et rece[dunt] mi[nuta] apostemata*, propter fumositates illuc transmissas; *fasti[dium] pa[tiuntur]*, vel propter defectum spirituum non excitantium virtutem desiderativam stomachi vel propter corruptos humores a quibus corrupte fumositates resolvuntur et pariunt in ore stomachi abhominationem et sic fastidium. Et *in corpore*[119] *vesci[ce] nascu[ntur]*: propter fumositates et non morantur que fiunt ex

ventositate, *illi enim empici fiunt*, id est, expuentes saniem. *Quibus hec sunt signa qui vero velo[cius] empi[ci] fiunt*: dixerat auctor superius quod apostematum determinatio fit per putredinem; apostematum posuerat determinationem et non putredinem, ideoque determinationem putredinis in (138vB) sinuat. Diceret aliquis que sunt signa per que possumus investigare determinationem putredinis: *utrum ex hiis que diximus*[120] [scilicet signis] *aliquid conti[gerit] consi[derabis] an spiritus sit fre[quens]*, id est, actio inspirandi et respirandi. Frequentia inspirandi et respirandi fit ex forti calore cum siccitate, aër attrahitur ad corpus, non potest fieri multa dilatatio per siccitatem; quod non potest fieri una vice suppletur in temporis vicissitudine. Et *spu[tum] cum tussi non de[ficiente]*: ex transmissione materiei per traceam arteriam offenditur spiritus et sic tussis, et quia continua est ebullitio materiei per calorem, continuo aliquid resolvitur a materia ut in olla bullienti videtur. Continuo spiritus offenditur et sic tussis indeficiens et dicitur tussis indeficiens non eo quod non possit deficere sed non de facili. Et *utrum cum ex caliditate amplior*[121] *fiat*: quia sepe, sepius ex conamine excreandi comprimuntur membra et apostematis fit compressio et maior solutio continuitatis et sic maior dolor. *In talibus rupturam apostematis ante diem vicesimum expectabis*: ebulliens namque materia per calorem ducitur ad saniem. *Tunc cibum appe[tunt]*: quia non generantur corrupte fumositates facientes abhominationem, neque adest defectus spirituum propter quos deficiat appetitus. Et *quos fe[bris] in die rupture dimi[serit] eos eva[suros] iudicabis*: quasi diceret ruptura apostematis alia fit per naturalem calorem, alia per accidentalem; per accidentalem homo moritur, per naturalem liberatur. Et *modicum est atque coniunctum quod egerunt modicum est*: per quod insinuatur nunc fortis perturbatio stomachi que pater est familias, *et coniunctum*, id est, medium inter solidum et liquidum. *Pus quod prohici[unt] album est*: propter fortitudinem naturalis caloris operantis ebullitionem et dealbationem, *et leve*, id est, continuum propter defectum ventositatis; et *per totum equale*, id est, in continuitate, nam in toto et in parte deficit ventositas. In toto et in parte materiei fortis et equalis fuit actio caloris naturalis, et *sine la[bore]*, id est, sine dolore per quod declaratur quod materia non sit valde incentiva, et *cum modica tussi*, propter paucitatem materiei (139rA) et propter abscentiam furiositatis quia furiosa materia etiam pauce[122] existens; *veniens ad tra[ceam] ar[teriam]* et eam excoriando inducit multam tussim. *Hu[iusmodi] in brevi sanantur*: quia propter emergentia indicat naturam esse fortem. *Prope hiis sunt*, id est, cito determinatio egritudinis fiet in istis ad bonum, *proxima signa*, id est, consimilia

[118] latere *Vat 44vB, et fortasse* uno latere *passim vice* uno laterum
[119] per corpus *vice* in corpore *Vat 45rA* 30.99 videtur *vice* utrum *Vat 45rA*

[120] *post* diximus *addit* scilicet signis *Vat 45rA*
[121] excreare amplius *vice* ex caliditate amplior *Vat 45rA*
[122] *fortasse* pauca *vice* pauce

habent signis predictis; *quos autem fe[bris in] apostematis rupturam non deserit*, propter fortitudinem accidentalis caloris. *Iam indicati et quasi furtiva materia postmodum invad[it]*, id est, insultat adversus naturam, materia furiosa videtur reprimi in ruptura apostematis sed fortiter postmodum fieri discursio materiei et collectio operatur quod est eius quia discoriat, et *affici[untur] siti*, pro successione, et *fastidio cibi*, pro corruptis fumositatibus et egerunt molle. Ecce tale stercus fit vi sinthomatis sed fit propter incontinentiam materiei, et ex eo quod accedit ad mollitiem. Et *pus quod iactat livet*, propter mortificationem, et *livet*,[123] propter adustionem, *vel flegmati admixtum*, propter cruditatem, *atque spumosum*: quia omnis spuma cum colore significante calorem furoris est inditium, cum colore significante frigiditatem indigestionem vel ventositatis insinuat presentiam. *Hiis signis [pertractatis] perituros non [dubitabis] qui vero quedam horum* inefficatoria et *non omnia habuerint mortem hii quidem moriuntur hii quidem in vita manebunt*: qui habuerint plura bona efficatoria.[124] *Utrique tamen difficilem exitum consequentur*: medici, quia ipsa confusa et pronostica sunt latentia, *hii tamen providenti*[125] *tuo iuditio discernentur*, id est, debent discerni.

31. [*Prognostics XVIII*] *Quibus peripleumoniacis et cetera*: auctor intendit assignare determinationem apostematis peripleurici quod dicitur primitivum per apostema derivativum, dicens *quibus peripleumoniacis post aurem*, id est, superius, *et infra*, id est, inferius, *apostema contingerit*, apostemate peripleumoniaco primitivo per apostema derivatum ad superiora *pu[tredinem] efficit*, ebulliens per calorem materia transit in putredinem, et *cum crepuerit fistulam parit*, id est, fluxum (139rB) saniei. Et *sic evadit*, dum expurgatur materia quod parit per fistulam perversum fluxum saniei indicat cotidie generatum pro mortificatione membri loca ista existentia in aure vel iuxta vel infra aurem intricata sunt et membrorum habentium copiam consimilium ut venarum et arteriarum et nervorum. Collectio apostematis fit ibi materiei unde pro nimia sensibilitate et discursu humorum sequitur dolor. Multi humores ibi transeunt et discurrunt et putrefaciunt membrum. De cetero ad illud membrum non fiet discursus sed ad superficiale vel continuum vel contiguum, ut sic paulatim in uno membro consequatur ut in alio unde fistulam parit. *Interest tua diligentia*, O medice, id est, studio tuo, diligentiam adhibere, et *secundum hec precepta perpendere*, id est, hec precepta investigare. *Quando fe[bris] permanet*: ponit auctor quedam signa bona et quedam mala et efficatoria bona quam mala unde eger saluti restituitur. Et primo mala quam bona: mala sunt febres permanere in superficie per apostematis perseverantiam, *do[lor]*

non dimi[nuitur], pro discursu ad loca valde sensibilia, et *sputum inconveni[ens]*, pro defectu temperati humoris, *egestio non est colerica*, id est, humorosa— ecce bona signa quia egestio est media inter liquidam et solidam, *neque livida*[126] *pro mortificatione urina modica*: ecce signum malum et ecce bonum, *cum ypostasi plurima*, id est, cotidie apparet ypostasis usque ad creticam sui determinationem que declarat perfectionem tercie digestionis in membris. Et si tertia, bona secunda et prima, et *alia cuncta signa bo[ni] sunt nuncia*, ut actio inspirandi et respirandi. *Tunc sub aure apostema futurum exspectabis*: quia natura fortis expulsiva viget in toto corpore et in cerebro et si forte illa materia sui fortitudine expellatur ad cerebrum natura fortis cerebri expulsiva expellit sub aure. *Sepius inna[scitur] hic apostema quibus dolor atque calor est in ypocondriis*: ut si materia colligatur in pulmone collecta in superioribus pennis pulmonis indicat se esse calidam, unde rapitur supra aurem, et quia cerebro vicinantur (139vA) mortem inducit. Collecta materia in inferioribus pulmonis indicat se esse frigidum unde attrahitur ad inferiora, colligitur sub aure, et quia non vicinatur cerebro non inducit mortem. *Quibus vero peripleumonicis ypo[condria] inferiora neque dolent [neque] calent*:[127] quia superiora dolent et inferiora ut penne *hiis apostema supra aurem nascitur*, quia apostema est calidum.

32. *Apostema et cetera*: non solum fit determinatio apostematis peripleumonici ex transmissione melancolici ad aures, sed ad pedes. Materia existens in pulmone per arteriam mittitur ad pedes et ibi facit apostema. *Melius in principio sputi proiectio*: nulla enim melior determinatio in peripleumonia quam proiectio sputi, et tunc precipue laudatur determinatio cum sputum rubeum mutatur in album pro nature fortitudine, *hiis signis certa salus denotatur*. Si quod reicitur non est ut oportet ut sit viscosum vel globatum, viride vel nigrum, *neque in urina ypostasi[s] timendum est ei membro cui apostema supervenit periculum*: quia dissipat [et] mortem inducit, vel supervenit ita inquisita pluribus, materia transducitur ad pedes vel ad aliud membrum et membrum humidum putrefaciunt et cadunt. *Quod idem apostema si evanuerit*: pro raptu sui ad superiora; *neque fe[bris] defecerit*, quod mortem inducit. *Plures ex hiis qui grandivi*[128] *sunt*, id est, grandis evi ut senes *peripleumoniaca collectione depereunt*: quia omnia conveniunt in frigiditate unde moriuntur ex prolixitate egritudinis. *Alii vero aliis collectionibus magis*, ut iuvenes pleuresi quia omnia conveniunt in acumine.

33. [*Prognostics XVIIII*] *Acutis fe[bribus] et cetera*: auctor in hoc loco intendit ponere collectionem materiei ad apostema provenientis[129] in renibus.

---

[123] iactant *vice* iactat; viret *vice* livet (secundum) *Vat 45rB*
[124] *vide 113 supra*
[125] prudenti *vice* providenti *Vat 45rB*

[126] liquida *vice* livida *Vat 45rB*
[127] *fortasse* calent *vice* inferiora
[128] *fortasse* grandaevi *vice* grandivi
[129] *fortasse* proveniens *vice* provenientis

Acutis febribus existentibus: per quod declaratur materia acuta quam commitatur febris acuta, *si dolor a lumbis*, id est, materia doloris; *transcenditur a renibus ad diafragma superius*, ubi est cor. Materia calida et sicca virtutem habet dissecatoriam et dissolu(139vB)toriam transit ab ignobilibus ad membra nobilia inducit pleuresim. Et *aliis tamen signis previsis:* noli esse promtus in iudicio tuo ut mortem patienti ascribas, ex quorum pluralitate vel paucitate iudicabis. Si videris plura signa bona, noli iudicare de morte; si plura mala iudica de morte. *Vescica dolens:* propter collectionem materiei ad apostema in vescica et cetera. Vescica frigidum membrum est, non posset ita dolere nisi materia colerica, *atque rigida*, id est, dura per siccitatem. Materia est calida et sicca et non calida et humida, febribus non deficientibus, quia materia non versa neque in saniem neque in sclirosim, *ma[lum] pronunciabis:* retinetur ibi cum non possit emi propter oppilationem que habet virtutem dissecandi unde periculum aducit. *Magis cum ve[ntris] strictura:* longaon in principio sui habet collimitantiam cum vescica, facto apostemate in ventre, comprimitur longaon, unde denegatur exitus superfluitatis prime digestionis et secunde. *Sed [si] supervenerit urina quasi pus*, id est, pulverulenta, *cum ypostasi*, cum multis humoribus, *do[lor] solvitur*, cessante causa cessabit effectus. *Si vero [urina] non sic fuerit* pulverulenta cum ypostasi et *ve[scica] non mollescit* et apostematis vescica non ducatur ad saniem, *neque fe[bris] deci[derit] mors in primo peryodo* particulari, scilicet in septimo die, quia utrumque retinetur et stercus et urina. *Adherit*[130] *hec autem morbi species pueris amplius a septimo anno usque ad vicesimum annum eve[nire] consu[evit]:* quia in eis viget calor et humiditas et meatuum constrictio unde per poros apertos dissoluta humiditas non potest educi sed redundat vescice, ibi colligitur et facit apostema in noviter, genitis non potest fieri apostema quia habent subtillissimam humiditatem et habilem ad consumptionem. In iuvenibus nequaquam quia ipsi habent crossam humiditatem resistentem calori et habent meatuum apertionem unde evaporaret.

PARTICULA TERTIA

34. (140rA) [*Prognostics* XX] *In febribus idem terminus et cetera:* hic tertie particule est principium, que ascribitur virtuti spirituali eo quod signa hic posita sumuntur secundum vigorem vel vitium virtutis spiritualis. Inchoat auctor a febre ex qua virtus spiritualis potissime leditur, quoniam vero in precedentibus dixerat egritudines alias determinari in septimo, alias in quattuordecimo, alias in vicesimo. Quia earum determinationes possunt esse ad mortem vel ad vitam ne aliquis putaret terminum fore prefixum ita ad salutem quod natura ad mortem removet, auctor di-

cens, *in febribus idem terminus*, id est, eadem dies, *quibusdam ad mortem quibusdam ad vitam*, positurus auctor signa spiritualia determinationum, ponit quedam generalia quibus terminum cognoscatur fieri ad salutem quibus ad mortem. Et primo ad salutem dicens, *in quibus fe[bribus] si cuncta signa bene precesserint*, id est, omnia signa salutifera appareant ut motus digestionis divisionis et similium, et *spes ma[li]*, id est, timor mali, *in quoquam*[131] *non adheserit*, id est, coherentiam non habuerit vel quod nullum malum signum apparet. Si hec appareant in die indicativa, *in die quarta*, scilicet indicativa respectu illius [in]verta,[132] scilicet per regulam quaternarie computationis; *aut prius*, id est, in die tercio indicativo, *terminum iudicabis*, id est, egritudo ad bonum terminabitur. Verbi gratia si in undecimo die hec signa appareant, in quartodecimo secundum quaternarium egritudo terminabitur, vel in tertiodecimo secundum ternarium ad salutem. Ponit auctor signa quibus egritudo terminetur ad malum, ut si in die cretico indicativo omnia signa mala appareant in die illius indicativo, vel quaternarium egritudo ad malum determinabitur, dicens, *in quibus vero si cuncta signa ma[la] prove[nerint] neque spes boni ulla affuerit in die quarta*, indicativa per quaternarium vel ante, id est, indicativa per ternarium, *mortem obibit*.[133] Et quia huius[modi] determinationes in diebus creticis consueverunt fieri de eis tractat, dicens, *primus* (140rB) *periodus*, scilicet, universalis; primus, videlicet vicennarius, hoc numero continetur periodus alius est universalis aut particularis. Universalis periodus continet particulares sex ut primus vicenarius continet quatuor, septem, undecim, quatuordecim, septemdecim et viginti. Hoc est *primus in quarto, secundus in septimo, tertius in undecimo, quartus in quartodecimo, quintus in septimodecimo, sextus in vigesimo*: qui numerus per quaternarium[134] augmentando in acuta egritudine usque in vigesimo die decurrit, secundus a primo vicennario, scilicet in quadragesimo. *Neque est computari in completo [numero] et cetera:* hic Ypocras tacite respondet oppositioni. Posset enim queri quare quartus decimus et vicesimoquartus iudicantur cretici cum natura pares sint, et secundum quod idem inquit in Anforismis que imparibus iudicantur discreta sunt et amica conversioni. Et cum septimana dicatur a septimo et tres septimane faciant viginti et unum diem quare tres septimane spatio viginti dierum terminantur. Ad quod auctor respondet dicens, *neque est compu[tari] in comple[to] numero dierum*, id est, per complementum ut *in* et *completum* sint due partes, *quemadmodum neque anni neque menses computantur* per completum. Sed debemus computare per incompletum *ad quorum formas*, similitudinem, *tres septimane spatio viginti dierum terminantur:* licet annus dicatur spatium tre-

---

[130] *fortasse* adheret *vice* adherit

[131] aliquo *vice* quoquam *Vat 45vB*
[132] inventa *vice* [in]verta *Vat 45vB*
[133] mortem habibit *Vat 45vB*
[134] ternarium *Vat 46rA*

centorum sexaginta et quinque dierum et mensis spatium viginti et novem dierum vel triginta, et sic de ceteris; tamen secundum astronomorum rationem veridicam annus est spatium in quo sol totum zodiacum distincte peragrat et hoc spatio trecentorum sexaginta et quinque dierum et sex horarum. Quare ergo disextilis annus fiat in quarto anno hec est ratio, quia cum in unoquoque anno excrescant sex hore, que sunt quarta pars unius diei, et in tribus annis excrescant octodecim, in quarto anno excrescentibus sex horis dies completur integer, unde ille annus fit bisextilis. Mensis est spatium viginti et novem dierum et duodecim horarum in quo spatio luna totum suum zodiacum (140rA) distincte peragrat. Sicut ergo nunc annus nunc mensis computatur incompleto numero dierum, sic nunc septimana debet computari incompleto numero dierum. Septimana enium spatium est sex dierum et sedecim horarum in quo spatio natura tres suos motus exequitur. Ter ergo sex faciunt octodecim, ter sedecim faciunt quadraginta et octo horas, quibus divisis per medium faciunt duos dies. Duobus ergo diebus additis ad octodecim erunt viginti et sic tres septimane viginti dierum spatio terminantur. *De hinc*, id est, secundum hanc, *augmenti rationem primus periodus*, scilicet universalis. *Evenit in vigesimo [die], secundus in quadragesimo, tertius in sexagesimo*: videtur tamen auctor sibi contrarius. Dicit enim in Anforismis, *acute egritudines et cetera*: dicimus ergo quod intellexit auctor de acutis simplicibus sine apostematibus, hic de acutis cum apostematibus, vel dicimus quod ibi intellexit de continuis et acutis ut de terciana continua et similibus, hic de continuis et non acutis ut continua quartana, et cetera, que usque ad sexagesimum diem explusionem differunt.

35. *In quibus valitudinibus et cetera*: superius posuit auctor varias determinationes apostematum ubi dixit quedam determinari in vigesimo, quedam in quadragesimo, quedam alia in sexagesimo. Nunc agit de quibusdam egritudinibus in quibus determinatio est tarda quod cognoscitur quia pronostica in iniciis sunt latentia. Hoc autem habet fieri ex caloris remissione, nature debilitate, materiei cruditate et compactione unde egritudo prolixa. Dicit ergo *in quibus valitudinibus*, id est, egritudinibus, *determinatio tarda est pronostica*, id est, signa salutis, *in iniciis sunt latentia, earum enim principia confusa sunt*: quando enim putamus esse augmentum adhuc adest egritudinis principium et sic in ceteris. Nulla ergo mortis vel vite emergunt indicia. *Ideo cautius vigilandum est*: si vis agnoscere si egritudo illa debeat per ternarium vel quaternarium terminari esto sollicitus et[135] videas in quibus diebus natura move(140vB)atur, utrum in terciis vel quartis. Et secundum quod videris pronosticorum eventum iudicabis utrum per ternarium vel quaternarium egritudo determinari debeat. *In singulis quaternis diebus*, id est, inventis per quaternarium; *studiosus intuendum*

est quod si feceris vix aut numquam[136] falleris et finis quartane, id est, quaternarie computationis, *est huiusmodi*, id est, in dignoscendo utilitatem habens utrum per quaternarium egritudo determinetur. Dixit superius quod si pronostica in principio sunt latentia, tarda adest determinatio, nu[n]c dicit *qui vero in brevi finiuntur facile cognoscuntur*, id est, pronostica a principio sunt manifesta; *differentia enim illarum est evidentissima*, quia ante fit determinatio ad salutem interdum ad pernitiem; dignoscitur enim determinatio ad mortem vel ad vitam per pronostica. Ponit auctor quedam signa per que future mortis vel vite habentur indicia, dicens, *evasuris quidem spiritus est suavis*, ex hoc enim vigor virtutis spiritualis denotatur. *Neque dolor aliquis*, qui significat venire, et *nocturna quies est naturalis*, id est, sompnus perfectam significat dispositionem cerebri et panniculorum eius. Et *cuncta signa reliqua boni ordinis ut diximus*, ut eger bene appetat et etiam sit compos sui, que omnia salutem demonstrant. Ponit auctor modo signa future mortis pronostica dicens, *morituris spiritus est anxius*, id est, inspiratio et respiratio frequens quod significat spiritualium succensionem, *turbatus animus*: turbata mens ex humorum perturbatione; *vigiliarum instantia*, ex dolore vel ex siccitate cerebri; et *omnis significatio mali est nuncia*, id est, future mortis previa, scilicet, ut non sit compos sui et cetera. Sed quoniam superius dixerat si appareant bona signa a principio salutem denunciant contrario mortem, ne generalitatis privilegium hec videatur sortiti, removet dicens *consi[derabis] igitur augmenti tempora usque ad statum*: nam si a principio appareant bona signa (141rA) debet providere ut si permaneant usque ad statum in bonitate, vel inmutentur ad malum de futura morte vel vita pronosticabis. *An sit ut supra disposuimus secundum hanc quoque rationem in pereuntibus cautus erit*: si enim omnia signa mala usque ad statum egritudinis perveniat crisim fieri ad mortem pronunciat.

36. [*Prognostics XXI*] *Si dolor in capite et cetera*: pronosticatur auctor circa cerebri apostema, ante enim apostema est in dura matre et dolor est acutus, quandoque in pia matre et dolor est acutior, quandoque in substantia cerebri et dolor est acutissimus. Dicit ergo *si dolor* est in capite acutissimus per quod notatur collectionem factam fore in substantia cerebri, et *cum fe[bre] fuerit*, quod significat materiam colericam esse in capite cuius acumine cerebrum dissipatur a quo omnia ducunt originem membra, mors sequitur. Et *si signum aliquod mortis appa[ruerit]*: unde spiritus anxietas mentis alienatio *mors cito aderit; et si signum aliud mali non affuerit*, scilicet, ut preter predicta signa ab Ypocrate posita, nullum mali appareat, et *dolor usque in vigesimum diem permanserit*, per quod insinuatur nature vigor potentis substinere dolorem adeo acutum; *neque fe[bris] abierit*, per quod insinuatur materiam non esse collectam ad apostema, sed vi

---

[135] *fortasse* ut *vice* et

[136] studiosus . . . aut vix aut nunquam *Vat 46rA*; *fortasse legendum est* studiose

nature ad aliquod aliud membrum inferius derivatur et per apostema determinatur. Vel, forti existente, natura novos ad inveniendo[s] meatus, materiam illam nondum ad apostema collectam per fluxum sanguinis e naribus evacuat. Ideo dicit *san[guinem] de na[ribus] exspec[tabis] aut aliquod apostema in inferioribus partibus corporis sed dolore adhuc retente*[137] *san[guinem] de na[ribus] et apostema sperabis*: quod significat materiam non esse confirmatam ad apostema sed per fluxum sanguinis evacuabitur unde ponit evidentiora signa. *Magis tamen:* per fluxum sanguinis materia expelletur. *Dolore frontem et timpora non derelinquente:* tunc enim materia venulis narium est vicina, citius ergo per fluxum sanguinis evacu(141rB)-abitur quia per aliud apostema determinetur. Ponit auctor adhuc signa per que potissime disnoscitur apostema cerebri determinari, aut per fluxum sanguinis, aut per apostema secundum etates, dicens *atque sanguinem*, id est, sanguinis fluxum sperabis; *plus [in] hiis quidem qui minus sunt triginta et quinque annorum*, id est, in adolescentibus in quibus natura fortis est multum et calor acutus. *Apostema vero in hiis*, sperabis, *que sunt anplioris etatis*, ut in senibus, in quibus vires sunt debiles et calor remissus unde natura non potest facere; facit materiam a nobilibus ad ignobilia a superioribus ad superiora[138] transducit et sic determinatio habet fieri per apostema inferius acutum.

37. [*Prognostics* XXII] *Aurium dolor et cetera:* auctor in hoc loco pronosticari intendit circa apostema aurium, dolor autem fit in auribus aliquando ex qualitate sola ut ex caliditate dissolvente, frigiditate constringente, humiditate relaxante, siccitate intercidente. Aliquando ex qualitate cum humore ad apostema collecto quia materia quedam obvolvitur crustula continua circa ipsam; ca[loris] fit ebullitio, ex ebullitione continua fit resolutio, unde continuo spiritus distemperantur et febris adest continua. Sed si fiat de frigido humore apostema febris erit continua et non acuta, **si** de calido erit continua et actua, permanens cum dolore aurium acuto. Dicit ergo *aurium do[lor] acutus:* per quod acuta materia declaratur, *cum acuta quidem fe[bre]:* quam materiam innuit calidam et furiosam et per malum;[139] *malum est quia exspectabis in eo alienationem et mortem:* materia enim cum sit calidissima et cerebro vicina sui acumine cerebri scindit substantiam unde mortem inducit, et eam inficiendo atque perturbando spiritum alienationem facit. *Gravem enim et mo[lestum] est:* et quia ex ipso apostemate quidam citius quidam tardius moriuntur. *Interest ergo tua*, id est, ad tuam utilitatem spectat, O medice, *omnia* apostemate *a principio perscrutari et attendere signa. Iuvenes qui sunt in hac passione:* id est, qui hac egritudine molestantur, *in septimo die vel prius*, id est, in quinta (141vA) *pereunt.* Iuvenes enim de natura complexionis et etatis calidi sunt et sicci et apostema

illud de calidissima et siccissima materia habet fieri, tum ergo dupplicat caloris actionem, scilicet complexionis, et etatis tum etiam acumine materiei natura defatigata succumbit. *Senes vero tardius pereunt:* scilicet ex hoc apostemate cum ex etate et complexione frigidi sunt et etiam materia in eis ex debilis caloris actione nequeat levigari, vicinam tamen mortem indicat, quod patet. *Quod fe[bres] et alie[natio] minus eis quam iuvenibus contingit:* propter caloris remissionem, unde in hiis non acumine materiei sed prolixitate mortem consuevit inducere. *Atque aures eorum*, id est, senum, *rumpuntur, et pus*, id est, putredinem *emittunt in senum tamen etate*, id est, in senectute, quia natura debilis est ex etatis prorietate dum sanies perfecte nequid expurgari; *valitudo*, id est, egritudo, *resurgit et interimit*,[140] temporis diuturnitate. *Iuvenes quoque antequam rumpatur apostema pereunt:* ex nimietate acuminis et furiositate materiei. Natura enim suo vigore tantum nequid tollerare acumen; quod apostema *si crepuerit*, id est, in iuvenibus, *et signum quodlibet boni apparuerit*, ut patiens non sit alienus a mente, scilicet compos sui, *aliquid boni sperabis*, id est, de futura salute, *materia enim de vi nature ad saniem ducitur et expurgabitur.*

38. [*Prognostics* XXIII] *Apostema in gutture et cetera:* agit auctor in hoc loco de apostemate gutturis quod habet fieri in branco et non de quinancia, ut quidam opinantur; huiusmodi autem apostema fit ex catarro, dum enim hu[mores] a capite ad guttur effluunt et precipue ad brancum sive antimeron, vel cum trameti cum[141] actione caloris obvolvuntur crustula et sic efficitur apostema. Dicatur ergo *apostema in gutture cum acuta fe[bre] ma[lum] est:* quia ex eo denegatur actio inspirandi et respirandi, aditus cibo et potui, et *si aliud mali signum ex predictis visum fuerit:* ut mentis insania (141vB) vel aliquod aliud, *mortale est.*

39. *Quinancia et cetera:* agit auctor in hoc loco de apostemate gutturis quod habet fieri in ysmon, in quodam scilicet folliculo, qui habet esse inter duo principia, scilicet inter traceam arteriam et ysophagum et diversa sortitur vocabula secundum variam positionem materiei. Si enim toto materia intus in ysmon colligitur inducit quinanciam, si tota extra squinanciam, si partim intus partim extra sinanciam. Licet omnes periculose sint: tamen quinancia omnibus periculosior est et inpossibile est aliquem de ea liberari nisi materia ad exteriora vertatur. Dum enim materia omnino in interioribus consistit constrigitur ysophagus, quo constricto cibo et potui denegatur aditus, constringitur etiam tracea arteria, qua constricta actio inspirandi et respirandi denegatur et sic sequitur subita suffocatio. Sinantia non est adeo periculosa et possibile est de ea patientem liberari nisi materia intus multa consistat et que manet exterius interiora petat. De squinantia omnes liberantur nisi materia intus con-

---

[137] superioribus partibus *Vat 46rB*; *fortasse* restante *vice* retente
[138] ad inferiora *Vat 46rB*
[139] permanentem *Vat 46vA*, *fortasse recte vice* per malum

[140] intermittit *Vat 46vA*
[141] *fortasse* trametico *vice* trameticum *sive* trameti cum

vertatur. Dicit ergo *squinancia*[142] *pessima et cito mortifera:* inter cetera apostemate que febre committantur nullum isto periculosius et mortalius, cum ex febre fortis fiat spiritualium consumptio et succensio, unde patiens multa indiget frigidi aëris attractione ad innatam distemperantiam tepescendam. Huiusmodi autem attractio nequit fieri, cum ex apostematis presentia in ismon et tracee arterie fiat constrictio, et fumositatum nulla exalatio, et sic suffocatio. *Que in gut[ture] non appa[ret]*: quod significat materiam omnino fore collectam in interioribus, *nec extat in cervice cum rubenti tumo[re]*, quia tota materia intus est; *do[lore] tamen acu[tissimo] exi[stente]*, per quod materiei acumen insinuatur; et *spiritu ortomie*, id est, rectionis. Cum enim materiei multitudo collecta est in ysmon tracea arteria comprimitur, unde libera nequit fieri inspiratio et respiratio, recte ergo morantur (142rA) ad liberiorem aëris attractionem et fumositatu[m] liberam exalationem, si enim ad collum convertantur multa fieret constrictio tracee arterie et sic suffocatio. *Vel mali spes in prima die suffocat aut secunda sive tertia vel quarta:* ultimum terminum ponit quam progredi nequeunt et ad quam vix aut nunquam deveniunt. Ponit modo de secunda specie scilicet de sinancia, dicens *altera huius mali*[143] *species est cum in gut[ture] apostema rubet*, quia materia partim intus, partim extra colligitur, *et ipsa mortifera est, tamen pigrior est:* ad interficiendum predicta vel pigrior, id est, magis durans in vita. Agit de tertia specie, dicens *tertia vero cum cervix et guttur rubent prioribus diuturnior est*, id est, diutius perseverans, et *nisi tumo[r] [ad] interiora*[144] *redierit*, per quod significaretur raptus materiei ad interiora, *spei omnino locus non deerit*, sperandum est enim de futura salute, et *si delituerit*, id est, cum apparet subito. *Non apparet tamen non in ipsa die cretica:* per quod significaretur materiam vi sinthomatis mitti ad interiora, *nec propter aluid apostema rubentem*, tumorem alio transduxerit per quod insinuatur materiam non esse derivatam inducendo apostema in interioribus, *neque putre[dinem] patiens expuerit*, per quod ostenditur materiam non esse ductam actione caloris ad saniem et nullatenus evacuari, *vel ad modicum* defecerit, per quod insinuatur materiam paulatim consumi, et *si do[lor] et alleviatio metitur requiem*, dum enim materia omnino mittitur ad interiora in ipso raptu substantia[145] egri videtur fieri alleviatio, dum tamen venit ad spiritualia suffocationem inducit. *Unde mortem vel iterationis labo[rem] promittit:* nam aliquando non est tanta materia ut suffocationem valeat inducere et spiritualium virtus fortis, dum enim materia ad se venientem repellit, ad pristinum locum deducit et ideo non in merito recidiva sequitur. *Bo[num] est autem tu[morem] et ruborem*

foris promittere:[146] cum materiei egressus declaretur a deteriora [ad exteriora]:[147] *quod si idem apostema intus lap[sum] fuerit ad pulmonem*, id est, apostematis materia; *pus ibi efficitur*, actione (142rB) caloris, *et amentem reddit:* quia de putrida materia putrida resolvitur fumositas, veniens ad cerebrum eius substantiam inficit et amentiam facit.

40. *Uvam tumidam et ru[bentem] et cetera:* superius auctor pronosticatus est circa apostema gule, nunc pronosticari intendit circa apostema uve, quoddam membrum a palato dependens in modum uberum mamillarum. Dicitur autem uva quia uve gerit similitudinem, quod enim est superius et palato continuum est et latum, quod vero inferius acutum, superius magno, inferius parvo foramine contentum. Hoc autem membrum a natura est destinatum ut cerebri superfluitates per ispum expurgentur; fuit autem angusto foramine inferius contentum ut superfluitates illuc venientes paulatim per excreationem expellerentur. Si esset largum hu[mor] repente distillaretur in multa quantitate ad spiritualia unde eorum fieret suffocatio, vel ideo a natura est dispositum ut aërem attractum depuraret, si vero pulverulentus attrahitur depuratur dum pulvis ipsius membri coheret substantie qui postea per excreationem sputo admixtus aducitur. In hoc autem membro sanguis quandoque ad apostema colligitur et uva redditur tumida, unde dolor sentitur infixivus, aliquando flegma naturaliter colligitur et uva est subtumida, albescit et dolor est extensivus. Interdum colera et tunc est crocea aut citrina et dolor adest pungitivus, quandoque melancolia et est terrei coloris et dolor adest generativus aut paucus aut nullus sentitur. Ponit autem Ypocrates dupplicem eius curam, quia aut nummo calido aureo est curanda, et desiccantibus speciebus, aut incisione, et quia suffocationis debemus evitare periculum, primo generalis precedat purgatio ut humoris diminuatur habundantia, detur etiam opiata et sic fiat incisio, tempore tamen favente et suffocationis periculo minime reluctante, ne tempus sit reumaticum. Dicit ergo *uvam tu[midam] et ru[bentem]*: per quod materia sanguinea declaratur, *incidere*, ferro, *timendum est*, quia sanies sequitur. Cum enim continuus fiat fluxus (142vA) per uvam et locus ille perforatus nequeat cicatrizari dum humores decurrentes in saniem convertuntur, patiens fit empicus, id est, saniem excreans, empima vero transit in ptisim; *vel san[guinis] fluxus ni[mius] se[quitur]*, dum propter incisionem emorrosagia sequitur, *la[borabis] igitur ad aliam curam confu[gere]*, id est, adustionem vel appositionem desiccantium, et *si ne[que] incisione sic effugere poteris et amplius crescit et livescit:* per hoc quod crescit materiei non significatur consumptio, per hoc quod livescit ipsius mortificatio, *et a palato quod heret subtiliatur*, quod significat materiam ponderosam et in inferiori parte collectam, *tunc incide*

---

[142] quinantia *Vat 46vA*
[143] huiusmodi *Vat 46vB*
[144] ad interiora *Vat 46vB*
[145] *fortasse* substantie *vice* substantia

[146] prominere *Vat 46vB*
[147] a deterioriis ad exteriora *Vat 46vB*

sed prius totum corpus curare festinabis, id est, purgare sicut predictum est; *tempore favente*, ne tempus sit reumaticum in quo fit maior fluxio; *et suffocationis timo[re] non reluc[tante]*, quia huiusmodi apostema commitatur febre subdit: *quorum fe[bris] si [per] modicum lente[scerit]*, per quod insinuatur aliquantula partis materiei consumptio; *neque signum fini[endi] egritudinis habuerit neque fe[bris] defectus in die cretico fuerit:* per quod declaratur materiam non esse consumptam et in multa quantitate esse collectam, *[et] iterationem egritudinis exspec[tabis]*, et quia calor desuffocatur, videtur febr[is] lentescere. Postmodum calor circa materiam ebullitionem praestantem de materia fit repletio predicte egritudinis fit iteratio. Curam apostematis uve et signa posuit pronostica, per que egritudinis significatur iteratio. Nunc ponit ipsius determinationem, scilicet per aliud apostema et non quodlibet sed per apostema iuncturarum. Ante enim natura est debilis, unde perfectam nequid celebrare crisim, sed quam potest operari operatur, materiam a nobilibus ad ignobilia transducit et maxime ad ea membra in quibus viget virtus attractiva propter motum, scilicet, ad articulos et iuncturas. In eis igitur dum materia actione caloris obvolvitur crustula efficit apostema et sic apostematis uve fit determinatio. *[Prognostics XXIIII]* Dicit ergo *quibus fe[bribus] permanet:* quod materiei significat presentiam circa quam calor continuam prestat ebullitionem et febris continue causa efficitur. *Neque labo[re] generantur:* quod significat materiei cruditatem et frigiditatem unde in egro non est tanta (142vB) anxietas; *neque uve multo do[lore] mo(lestantur]*, quod significat materiei cruditatem et compactionem in qua calor parvam prestando ebullitionem parvam inducit continuitatis solutionem. *Hiis apostema est futurum in iuncturam tamen parcium inferiorum:* propter sui gravitatem qua movetur inferius; *transactis vero viginti diebus post fe[brem]*, id est, post febris principium, cum enim materia sit compacta, longum tempus expostulat ad sui digestionem. Nunc auctor in quibis etatibus hiis[148] apostematis fiat determinatio et minus habeat provenire, dicens hoc idem apostema in iuncturis inferiorum membrorum. *Minus evenit illis quorum etas inferior est a quadragesimoquinto anno:* quia cum in eis calor fit[149] fortis aut materia calore consumitur, aut eius actione ad saniem ducitur, aut vigore nature omnino ad alia membra transducitur, unde statim febris decidit. *Sed quibus etas est prolixior*, ut in senibus, *apostema fit*, id est, huiusmodi apostematis determinatio febribus manentibus: hoc ideo fit cum enim in ipsis natura sit valde debilis et calor remissus multe superfluitates in eis generantur que morbi augmentant materiam, unde pre nimia natura debilitate licet pars materiei ad iuncturas ossium transmittatur et ad apostema colligatur, pars tamen materiei que

remanet adhuc febrem sufficit inducere unde febris permanet.

41. *Febribus et cetera:* Ypocras secundum varium parosismum egritudinis pronosticari intendit. Paroxismus dicitur exacerbatio, paroxismus aut est ordinatus aut inordinatus: ordinatus est ille quando consueto[150] et egrum invadit accessio ut tercia de tercio in tercium. Inordinatus est ille quando non secundum statutum ter febris affligit patientem si nunc de tertio in tercium, nunc de quarto in quartum, nunc de quinto in quintum et sic de ceteris. Hoc autem significat diversorum humorum dominium unde nunc putrescit colera et suam actionem inducit, nunc flegma, nunc melancolia. Dicit ergo *fe[bribus] inordi[nate] vagantibus*, que dicuntur erratice seu planetice: *quartane sunt future, melancolicus* enim humor ceteris compactior ultimo aliis humoribus affligit. Colera enim altera sui qualitate putrefactioni resistens longum tempus (143rA) expostulat ad sui digestionem unde aliis humoribus consumptis, erratica in quartana[m] mutatur vel quia colera actione caloris adustam quartanam facit. *Certius tamen circa autumpnum:* tunc enim melancolici humoris multa fit generatio ex temporis furiositate, *et sicut illis quos diximus*, id est, in senibus, *apostema oritur sic qui trigesimumquintum annum preterierint[151] quartanarii efficiuntur:* propter concordiam etatis frigide et sicce, tales enim senes sunt.

42. *Apostematum et cetera:* ultimo loco Ypocras quandam ponit generalem apostematis doctrinam, dicens *omne apostema magis fit in yeme:* omnis apostematis maneries, *quam in ceteris temporibus:* hoc universale signum omne comprehendit hic genera singulorum et non singula generum. Quia et sanguineum et colericum et melancolicum, tamen videtur plane contrarium, quia cum colera in multa quantitate generetur in estate in epate et tunc superhabundet, quia apostema colericum magis deberet fieri in estate quam in yeme, ad quod dicimus quia in estate quamvis generetur multa colera non potest in unum locum coadunari nec concludi, quia propter calorem aëris aperientem poros colera in fumum resoluta exalat. In yeme vero, quamvis in pauca quantitate colera generetur pro nimia frigiditate, pori constringuntur, unde superfluitates colerice retente per eandem habentem motum ad centrum in unum locum cumulantur et cuticula obvolute apostema confitiunt. Non tamen qualibet parte corporis sed in spiritualibus, dum ea tanquam frigida et debilia superfluitates mittuntur. Iterum quamvis in autumpno magis de melancolia generetur, tamen propter vicinitatem estatis calor conservatur in aëre unde, poris apertis, fumositates exalant quod non fit in yeme. Sanguineum apostema magis in yeme propter multas fumositates generatas, inficientes ipsum sanguinem quam in vere in quo purus sanguis generatur. Vel aliter apostema aliud est primitivum

---

[148] *fortasse* huius *vice* hiis

[149] *fortasse* sit *vice* fit; quadragesimo *legitur etiam Vat 47rA*

[150] consuete *vice* consueto it *Vat 47rA*

[151] pretereunt *Vat 47rA vice* preterierint

et aliud derivatum, quod ex alio apostemate derivatur ut apostema sub aure quod fit ex pleumonia, ut diximus. Omne igitur apostema derivatum magis (143rB) fit in yeme quam in ceteris temporibus. Tunc enim multe superfluitates generantur, in unum locum collecte, ponderositate substantie mittuntur ad alias partes et ad apostema colliguntur. *Et amplius moratur:* propter multitudinem materiei, *et si sana[tur] non reci[procatur]*: quidam volunt dicere quia natura tunc est fortis, unde postquam apostema ducitur ad saniem materia omnino evacuatur, membrum aut forte existens prohibet materiei discursum unde non fit recidiva. In aliis vero temporibus quia membra sunt debilia, expurgata materia fluenti humori fit contradictio ideo reciprocatio. Vel aliter, in estate propter siccitatem materia apostematis condempsatur, unde mortificatur calore aut postmodum in ipsam agentem dissolvitur et sic apostema reciprocatur. Sed in yeme frigide aëris calor intercluditur ciuus actione materia ad saniem deducitur, ducta vigore nature evacuatur quare non sequitur recidiva. *Quibus adsunt fe[bres] et cetera:* positis signis diversitatum apostematum, ponit signa febrium per que egritudines et maxime interpolatas, ut pote tercinam, per vomitum determinari pronosticabis, dicens *quibus adsunt fe[bres] non mortifere:* febres non mortifere dicuntur interpolete[152] respectu continuarum in quibus nunquam per acumen afflictionis natura succumbit. Vel dicuntur non mortifere in quibus nulla mortis pronostica apparere videtur, aut quod de terciana nil ad eius intentionem spectet cum eius intentio sit circa acutas egritudines. Respondentes quod hic circa acutas pronosticatur, nam terciana alia vera, alia notha. Vera est in qua omnia particularia vel eorum plura cum naturalis materiei conveniunt proprietatibus, non vera in qua omnia particularia vel eorum plura a naturalis materiei discrepant proprietatibus, vel que fit de innaturali materia. Hic ergo cum agat de terciana non de qualibet agit, sed de vera, de acuta passio, dicitur,[153] et cita mortifera iudicatur, nisi quia est interpolata et brevis egritudo in qua cum virtus in actione debilitetur in die quietis natura confortatur. Brevis est quia cum fiat (143vA) de materia calida et sicca per caliditatem et siccitatem dissolvitur materia et dissoluta cito consumitur, unde in Anforismis terciana vera in septem periodis iudicatur longissima. Et *testatur do[lor] in capite:* quod significat materiam colericam et calori obedientem que levis est, unde in fumum resoluta petit cerebrum et inducit dolorem cerebri continuitate soluta. *Et pa[tientes] ante se putant tanquam muscas volare:*[154] dum enim materia in ore stomachi consistit liberos habens meatus et rectos, liberumque progressum ad superiora digestioni apta existens calore augente in ea in multum resolvitur fumum, qui dum mittitur ad anteriorem cellulam capitis spiritum visi-

bilem inficit, unde [si] fuerit rotunda talem spiritum representat forma, si quidem subtilis et oblonga talia spiritum representant corpuscula, et sic decet. *Aut aliqua nigra:* hoc autem significat maiorem actionem caloris circa materiam unde dum in fumum resolvitur actione caloris aduritur et denigratur, et sic spiritum inficiens nigrum ei representat colorem. Ponit etiam eius evidentius signum. *Et si dolor in vitalibus superve-[nerit]*: vita[lia] dicuntur spiritualia dum ergo quasi usque ad os stomachi impellitur propter multam ipsius ebullitionem, ex ea spiritualia comprimuntur, et sic dolor eorum signis hiis fientibus.[155] *Rubeam coleram vomituros sperabis:* adhuc addit signum evidentius, et *si frigus,* id est, rigor *affuerit,* id est, rigor provenit ex materia calida veniente ad os stomachi que pungendo et mordicando rigorem inducit. Et *in ypoc[ondriis] frigus sentitur:* quod significat materiei raptum ad os stomachi, sicut ergo sui presentia inferiora calefiebant sic sui abscentia infrig[i]dantur. *Certiorem et subitum vomitum sperabis:* (143vB) adhuc addit certitudinem, *et si cibum quem accipiunt reiciunt,* cum materia sit in ore stomachi propter caloris prestantem ebullitionem, cibaria ad exteriora expelluntur. Ponit auctor signa per que cita vel tarda crisis disgnoscatur, dicens *quibus dolor fit in capite a primordio fe[bris]*: per quod materiei aptitudo ad digestionem declaratur unde a principio caloris actione potest solvi. *In quarta et quinta die dolor augetur:* quia cum declaretur[156] augmentum fidei[157] succedit status in septima evadunt quia natura fortis materiam digestioni aptam expellit et crisis fit ad salutem. *Quibus vero in die tercia cepit dolor,* quia significat materiam minus calori obedientem. *Crescit usque in quintam et septimam:*[158] dolor per quod augmentum significatur, *et finitur in nona vel undecima,* si dolor crescat usque in quartam finitur in nona, si usque in septimam in undecima fiet crisis vel prolixior fiet crisis, unde dicit *est etiam ubi contingat,* dolorem scilicet incipere, fiet *in quinta die,* quod significat materiei ineptiam ad digestionem in illis scilicet *quorum urina priori*[159] *similis est,* id est, rubea cum ypostasi sibi simili, quod significat materiei cruditatem et morbi diuturnitatem,[160] vel cum ypostasi alba continua et equali et in fundo tunc prolongatur status quia *in quartadecima die liberantur,* id est, crisis fit ad salutem. Oportet ergo quod transeat undecimam diem et fiat computatio per quaternarium. *Que diximus terianariis eve[niunt] equaliter viris et mulieribus:* non modo eventus sed ipsum eventum insinuat. *Iunioribus,* id est, iuvenibus, *hec eveniunt in febribus diuturnis:* respectu vere terciane ut in sinocha et similibus. *In veris quoque tercianis:* in quibus omnia conveniunt cum

---

[152] *fortasse* interpolate *vice* interpolete
[153] sed de vera quia acuta passio dicitur *Vat 47rB*
[154] volitare *Vat 47rB*

[155] scientibus *Vat 47vA*
[156] dum declaretur *Vat 47vA*
[157] *fortasse* febri *vice* fidei
[158] quartam et septimam *Vat 47vA*
[159] natura priori *Vat 47vA*
[160] undecima dies *Vat 47vA*

proprietate materiei, quia calidi et sicci sunt, ut materia et omnia particularia vel eorum plura cum proprietatibus materiei conveniunt. Superius auctor posuit signa determinationis febris per vomitum, nu[n]c ponit signa futuri fluxus sanguinis, aliquando enim sanguis putrescit in venis inferioribus sub ypocondriis, unde vi nature materia sanguinea expellitur ad superiora et venulas narium abrumpendo per fluxum sanguinis evacuatur. Dicit ergo *in febribus si est dolor* (144rA) *capitis:* quod significat presentiam humoris et ventositatis in cerebro eius, miringas extendentis, unde fit dolor. *Neque ante oculos nigroribus quibuslibet apparentibus:* quod significat abscentiam colerici humoris adusti vel melancolici, unde fiet determinatio per vomitum, sed *veluti* [flamma] *lampadibus,* quod significat materiam fore sanguineam a qua fumus resolutus sibi similia corpora representat. Et *sub ypo[condria] dextra seu sinistra sunt tetani,*[161] id est, tensiones, quod significat materiam sanguineam impelli usque ad superiora unde venule extenduntur, et ypocondria, *sine dolore,* quod significat sanguinem ad apostema non esse collectum, quia tunc sui ponderositate ad superiora non ascenderet, *hiis sanguinis fluxurus est de naribus sicut predictum est.*

43. *Spasmus vero et cetera:* pronosticatur auctor circa spasmum ostendens in quibus etatibus maxime proveniat. Est autem spasmus contractio vel extensio nervorum seu lacertorum tocius corporis ex repletione ex inanitione seu ex frigiditate proveniens. Nervi enim repleti contrahuntur in longum distrahuntur in latum unde fit spasmus tunc interdum exsiccantur arefiunt, arefacti contrahuntur, dum contrahuntur nervi contrahuntur membra quibus sunt alligati et sic fit spasmus ex inanitione. Interdum frigiditas habendo motum ad centrum incurtationis membra contrahit et incurtat unde spasmus ex frigiditate. Quidam litteram istam spasmo ex repletione assignant, dicentes, *spasmus contingit pueris in acuta fe[bre],* id est, ex acumine febrilis caloris, cum enim in eis multa superhabundet humiditas calore dissolut[a], replet nervos et fit spasmus ex repletione. *Maxime vero si ve[ntrem] constrictum habeant:* quia significat retentionem superfluitatum unde maior repletio; *et vigilent,*[162] propter nimium dolorem inductum ex repletione et extensione; et *expavescant,* propter diversas yma(144rB)ginationes cerebro inductas ex diversorum humorum habundantia et *planga[n]t,*[163] propter humiditatem multam contentam in cerebro que partim missa ad oculos inducit lacrimas. *Et colores varii fiant*[164] secundum diversorum humorum dominium; *ut modo citri[ni],* ex habundantia colere, modo rubei ex habundantia sanguinis, *modo lividi,* ex habundantia mel-

ancolie, *modo viridea fia[n]t*[165] propter adustionem. *Hec eveniunt p[ueris] usque in septem annos,* donec multa est in eis substantialis humiditas. Dicimus autem finem legere, ut frequens littera demonstrat; de spasmo enim ex inanitione debet legi, cum enim in pueris humiditas liquida sit dissolutioni et consumptioni apta consueta substantiali humiditate nervorum arefiunt, arefacti contrahuntur. Ventris etiam constipatio ex intensione siccitatis provenit feces desiccantis. Vigiliarum instantia et timor ex caloris acumine consumentis et humoris adurentis habet provenire, nam dum nigra fumositas resolvitur et cerebrum petit spiritum inficiens timorem prestat. Non est mirum si timeant, quia causam timoris secum portant, quod plangunt de dissolutione substantialis humiditatis est cerebri, que actione caloris dissoluta in humores distillant et egredientes per oculos lacrimas producunt.[166] Variatio colorum ex varietate actionis calor[is] emergit, dum ergo colera resolvitur fit color citrinus, dum sanguis rubeus, dum melancolia lividus, dum etiam mala fit humorum adustio viridis color consurgit. Et eveniunt ista pueris usque in septem annos donec humiditas dissolutioni et consumptioni est habilis. *Maioribus et p[ueris],* id est, iuvenibus spas[mus] *non contingit,* ex inanitione. *In febribus nisi magnis existentibus infirmitatibus aut frenesi:*[167] nam cum in eis sit compacta humiditas non, nisi magna caloris et siccitatis actione, potest consumi, unde in eis spa[s]mus ex inanitione non evenit.

44. Operi suo auctor finem impositurus ammonet (144rA) medicum ut in signorum cognitione non sit negligens sive sint future mortis pronostica sive future vite. Ex altero namque laudem consequitur dum egrum saluti restituit quem mortis urget metus quem dolor excruciat infinitus; ex altero gloriam, dum finem morituro imponit et prorium finem consequitur. Ideoque in signis providendis in etate qualibet negligens non existat. Comparans vires egri ad vires egritudinis, comparans signorum bonitatem ad ipsorum malitiam, dicens *interest ergo tua,* id est, ad tuam utilitatem et diligentiam spectat, O medice, *ut multo studio pereuntes et evasuros sive pueros sive iuvenes discernas nec*[168] *in qualibet egritudinum,* id est, aliqua, *te negligenter offeras:* ammonet nos auctor ut in qualibet egritudine tam brevi quam longa, tam gravi quam levi, medicus se non offerat negligentem ut securus de signis possit mortem vel vitam predicere. [*Prognostics* XXV] *Honestum quoque illi est qui huic salutem promittit illi vero valet mortem pronunciare et in brevi et prolixa egritudine et omnes significationes,* id est, omnia signa ut diximus disnoscere et equa ratione perpendere atque vires eorum conferre ut predictum est. *Cautius tamen hec in urinis et sputis facere:* per ea namque dispositio

---

[161] sub ypocondriis ad dextra et sinistra sunt tensiones et tumores et tetani *Vat 47vA*
[162] vigilant *Vat 47vB*
[163] plangunt *Vat 47vB*
[164] variant *vice* varii fiant *Vat 47vB*

[165] fiunt *Vat 47vB*
[166] distillat . . . producit *Vat 47vB*
[167] ut frenesis *vice* aut frenesi *Vat 47vB*
[168] ne *vice* nec *Vat 47vB*

epatis et viarum urinalium, per sputum spiritualium. *Et hec mea doctrina est in acutis passionibus*, id est, hec predicta in acutis attenduntur.   Posuit signa que in acutis attenduntur, nunc ponit signa que in interpolatis attenduntur, dicens *nec etiam [in] epidimicis id est longis*, passionibus, *ut in cancro et similibus periculis torpeant.*   Et instituit que sunt attendenda dicens, *tempora presentesque morbos attendas*, id est, presentium morborum tempora, scilicet principium, augmentum, statum et declinationem ut competentem scias adhibere modum curationis.   Ne aliquis putaret quod egritudines ita provenirent in uno tempore quod non alio, dicit: *Scito omnes valitudines omnibus anni* (144vB) *temporibus posse evenire:* ut omnes comprehendant singulorum genera et non singula generum ut dicatur omnes egritudines, id est, doloribus, *tamen quasdam magis quibusdam evenire:* nam terciana magis in estate, quartana in autumpno, cotidiana in yeme. Ammonet tamen nos ut circa signorum noticiam medicus insistat, dicens *quarum signa ma[la] sunt malas esse quarum vero bo[na] e contrario se habere*, id est,

bonas esse, videtur tamen contrarium aliquam egritudinem bonam dici; dicitur tamen bona, id est, non pernecabilis ad necessitatem tamen et proba[bi]litatem.   Inducendam in sua doctrina dicit ea se fore expertum in tribus paribus mundi dicens, *ad huc significationes que diximus in Ethiopia septentrione et Esperia*, id est, in Yspania; *experti sumus nec aliqua desperatio te perturbet quia locupletius quam existimes arridebit tibi signorum series*, id est, favorabilis apparet series, *si[c]ut novimus rationi invigiles;* et quia Ypocras, quasi prophetico spiritu noverat quosdam pseudomedicos futuros, ne medicum falsis illorum preceptionibus adhereret, ipsius preceptiones dimittendo, subinfert, *neque velis te ad alias preceptiones*, id est, precepta, et *alias egritudines*, id es, egritudinum signa, *diffundere quia quecumque egritudines terminantur nostro numero*, id est, per ternarium sive per quaternarium, *nostro quoque exposito ordine preceptorum*, id est, earum determinationis[169] noticiam per meam, O medice, doctrinam habebis.

---

[169] determinationem *Vat 48rA*

MAURUS OF SALERNO:
COMMENTARY ON THE PROGNOSTICS OF HIPPOCRATES

PREFACE

1. The dazzling splendor of the *Prognostics* of Hippocrates, by exploring and illuminating completely the secret storehouses of the mind, reveals certain hidden signs of the human organism and brings order to those subjects concerning which Hippocrates made observations during a lifetime of experience in medical practice. For he probed into the threefold nature of matter, a subject with which knowledge in general is concerned, and the significance of which seems in some measure to surpass all others. Because the perfect state of the body is also of a threefold nature and triple causation, he correspondingly reveals his knowledge in three stages, and by so doing casts light on many obscure problems (1). Borrowing whatever was appropriate, Hippocrates excerpted from his other writings an individual book devoted exclusively to signs, and we have now begun the study of this text (2).

In the brief foreword are found the following subjects: the content and plan of the work, the motive for writing it, its underlying usefulness, its subdivisions, an outline of the discussion and the book's title (3). The subjects are threefold, namely, the body's form, action, and excretions, and indeed, every sign is derived either from the body's form, action, or excretions. Our author's purpose is to point out, by means of this triad, the certainty of those signs by which we may judge, especially in acute and very acute diseases, the approach of death or the length of life to be expected.

The motive which inspired the work was the rashness or contrariety of the Empirics and Methodists, who through their inattention to signs and causes converted brief illnesses into lengthy ones, and curable illnesses into incurable. His design was also to emphasize the excellence of the human body, and for this very purpose, he composed not only this work but many others. This book is useful in teaching us to review the patient's past history, to appraise his present state and to anticipate future developments. It is intended for use in actual practice, because through it we may acquire a thorough knowledge of signs. Now from actual practice we progress to medicine, from medicine to physic, from physic to theory, and from theory we may contemplate philosophy (4).

The work itself is divided into three parts because of the three virtues, the first being the animal, the second the natural, and the third the spiritual. An outline of the discussion is as follows: the author opens with a brief statement in which he invites the logical physician to undertake the study of this useful and honorable profession through a survey of universals and particulars. He then proceeds according to this plan and discusses in the first part those topics which are to be considered in relation to the strength or weakness of the animal virtue; in the second part those relating to the natural virtue; and in the third part those relating to the spiritual virtue (5).

The title reads *Here begins the Book of the Prognostics*: although in general he discusses present as well as past signs, the book nevertheless treats more fully of prognostic signs, and by the rule of peer among peers, prognostic signs are held in higher esteem than signs of the past or present. For, as Galen puts it, although past signs are very useful, and present signs are even more so, yet prognostic signs are by far the most useful (6). This is obvious, because we may defer or entirely avert future events, but we can in no way alter past events as they either did or did not occur. Again he may have called the book *The Prognostics* because the expression "prognostic sign" had for the ancients an implication of no greater weight than any other sign, and we note in the *Tegni* that Galen considers all signs to be quite useful in prognosis, including those already observed in the past and during the present.

2. *Every one and so forth*: in this work Hippocrates omits a lengthy introduction, thus setting a good example for writers who embellish their works with a host of testimonials. This also makes the reader more docile, benevolent, and attentive: docile, because he states that the reader will know the past, present, and future course of individual illnesses; benevolent, because he emphasizes the usefulness of the work; and attentive, because he asserts that through the art of medicine, and especially through this book, the physician will acquire for himself and for his colleagues great praise and glory (7). Glory, by recalling the past, demonstrating the present, and predicting the future; praise, because he restores to health a sufferer oppressed by the fear of death and tortured by unceasing pain. He will also acquire a a host of friends, because by healing one person he relieves all those who were tormented by that person's pain. *Everyone who seeks the pleasure or glory of medical science* (8): study is the ardent application of the mind to any subject which an individual pursues with great zeal, whereas glory implies repeated praise and public recognition, *should frame his reasoning according to the rules of prudent men*, or philosophers, *as applied to illness*. For even illness may be considered an aspect of health because we learn from

illness whether nature prevails over disease or disease over nature. Illness is also termed an aspect of health to imply the very end of life, as was done by the ancient writers; or it is called an aspect of health in the contrary sense, not because it brings health but because it takes health away. By recalling *the past*, demonstrating *the present*, and predicting *the future*, the physician becomes informed about the sick man and reveals facts to him which he scarcely realized about himself. Hippocrates praises prognosis most highly, because if to demonstrate the present is greater than to remember the past, to predict the future must be still greater. If the physician, unaided, reveals and explains to a patient those points about his medical history which should be evident, the patient will have greater confidence in what is being done for his health, and his eagerness to cooperate will enhance the effectiveness of treatment.

The purpose for which medicine exists is praiseworthy, although the physician's purpose differs from the patient's. It is the physician's duty to preserve, protect and cure; the patient's to be cured and protected. The physician does not always attain this end, and, as Boethius remarks, "the physician will not always cure, nor the orator always persuade, nor the sophist always beguile" (**9**), but if the physician has overlooked none of the various possibilities we shall consider that he has discharged his obligations very well. Another precept which the physician must always observe is that he should treat only those who are capable of being cured and relinquish his efforts when prognostic signs indicate that the case is hopeless, *for as the author says, each case must be judged individually, and it is obviously impossible to cure all the sick* (**10**). The physician must therefore not expect that a definite result will invariably follow his treatment, for this does not happen, *and if all patients could be cured, a physician would be called not a prophet but a god*, that is, more noble than a prophet, and *truly divine*.

Although it is true that some die suddenly through the violence of a disease, that is, by an acute exacerbation, a patient may die in one of two ways, from the violence of the disease itself or from the viscosity of undigested matter impacted in the viscera (**11**). Here the "vis" refers to "viscosity," but when he speaks of "violence," he also refers to the excessive strength of the treatment. Death may occur naturally or by accident, a natural death being one which has a predetermined end, of which we may say that we have correctly estimated the terminal date beyond which the illness could not continue; an accidental death is one whose occurrence we might possibly have been able to prevent. *Some die before the physician arrives or live on scarcely for a day*, this is a death by accident. *It is therefore useful for the practitioner*, and pertains to the worth of his art, *to estimate whether the sick man's strength and the violence of the disease are well balanced.*

The physician skilled in diagnosis strives to learn, by study of the signs, the evolving trend towards life or death.

There is indeed something divine about prognosis and some say that a hidden sign is a heavenly sign, for if a physician could know definitely whether the outcome were to be life or death he could quickly predict the final result. Others suggest that our author really encourages us here to a study of astronomy through which we may recognize the present, past, and future, and indeed this is a heavenly science *with which* certainly the physician ought to have some personal familiarity (**12**), *and because of his remarkable foresight he will be greatly admired*, because through such foresight he may study general tendencies toward life and death, *and decide whether any immediate danger exists which can in any way be warded off*. This foresight is connected with the physician's *ability to respond either in counteracting a disease or in making the patient more comfortable* by moderating its severity, because even if a patient cannot be freed from death, the physician must nevertheless do everything in his power to make the illness seem lighter. *And if he announces in advance who will die and who will recover, he will avoid censure and deserve much praise*, because it reflects on his skill in the art to be able to predict death for those who will die and health for those who will recover (**13**).

SECTION ONE

3. [*Prognostics I*] *He ought and so forth*: having completed his prefatory remarks, Hippocrates now returns to his announced purpose, namely, to discuss the signs in acute diseases. This is obvious from the contents of the work where he states that the physician must concern himself first with acute illnesses. This is also the theme of the first section we assign to the animal virtue, not because it arises in the brain which is the seat of the animal virtue, but because in acute diseases it is there that signs are to be found which may prove useful and which will vary according to the strength or weakness of the animal virtue. He here discusses acute and very acute diseases whose critical periods are often difficult to determine. Moreover, Constantinus in his book *On Fever* provides a classification of nine favorable and unfavorable signs (**14**).

The first favorable sign is the sick man's strength and resolution to sustain his illness, the contrary is his weakness or inability to do so. The second favorable sign is ease of motion of the body and its various members, even within moderate limits; the contrary is any inertness of the entire body and its various members. The third favorable sign is for the patient's countenance to be similar to that in health; the contrary is an appearance dissimilar to that in health. The fourth favorable sign is soundness of mind and regular elimination; the contrary sign is an unsound mind and irregularity of elimination. The fifth favorable sign is regularity of sleep; the contrary is irregularity of sleep. The sixth favorable sign is ease of breathing, that is, of inspiration and expiration; the contrary is difficulty in breathing. In this connection, rapid breathing implies that parts near the diaphragm are involved in the disease. The seventh favorable sign is regularity of the pulse; its contrary is irregularity. The eighth favorable sign is strength of the innate heat at the point of coction of matter added to good strength of the digestive apparatus; the contrary is weakness of innate heat at the point of coction of matter and weakness of the digestive apparatus. The ninth favorable sign is adequate expulsion of waste matter through the regular channels; the contrary is inadequate expulsion of such matter through the regular channels.

When occasionally the physician erroneously promises a certain return of health to a dying man, he does not deserve to be censured, but in order to avoid similar complaints in other cases [*Prognostics II*] *he should first be careful to study the face in every acute illness.* As we stated previously, all indications are derived from the body's appearance, from observed signs and from excreted residues. Because these signs are more worthy of our attention, he first discusses the signs revealed by the body's form. Now three factors determine an object's Nature: its Maker, its substance, and its form. Of these, the Maker is manifestly primordial and more worthy than the others, and it is from the One that the others derive their causal origin. The second is clearly substance, from which are derived matter and subject, and from which in turn there is no further subdivision as to number or variety. Forms being imposed on matter, he separated these by turns and arranged them in classes under certain genera of things (**15**). In discussing signs derived from the body's appearance, he speaks first of those derived from the appearance of the face, either because the face is the first part seen by observers, or because it has a tender and delicate substance which becomes altered and tinged with color by the slightest excess of any quality or by the slightest harmful humor, as may be noted in jaundice when a greenish color appears in the face before any other part of the body (**16**). Perhaps there is still another reason, namely, that the most potent factors influencing the individual's state and form, in fact life itself and the senses, can both be best observed in the face, the former through inspiration and expiration, the latter because the five senses are located there (**17**).

First notice the patient's appearance, for in this manner you may decide *whether it resembles his appearance in health,* and observe whether indeed the patient has changed greatly from his earlier condition (**18**). From this the sick man's strength to sustain the power of the disease may be ascertained; on the other hand, some sick people look healthy although they suffer pleurisy or pneumonia, but because of interference with respiration, they become flushed on the side of the disease (**19**). For that reason he inquires whether *the patient resembles his normal self,* that is, if he had been phlegmatic or melancholic during health, he should appear pale during illness, but if he had been of a ruddy complexion when well he should be proportionately so during illness. It is encouraging if these two favorable signs are present, one indicating that the features are similar to those in health, the other, an unchanged complexion, being the second favorable sign (**20**).

It is a bad sign if the features of the patient are dissimilar from those in health, or if through weakness the sick man lacks power to bear up under his illness. These signs are very bad, and one might add that there are other signs denoting evil which may be observed in the face, such as *if the nose becomes sharp.* Sharpness of the nostrils is an indication that accidental heat has consumed the nostrils' essential moisture, even though the nostrils share in some natural moisture through their own discharge; or if *the eyes are sunken,* either because an excess of accidental heat has consumed and dissolved the moisture of the eyes, or from constriction of the breathing apparatus. When intrinsic moisture is consumed in the lung the nerves become contracted, and because the nerves of the lung have a connection with the eyes the latter are also retracted, and appear sunken, for just as the eyes bulge out in hanged men, so in those who are suffocated the eyes are drawn inward.

If *the temples are sunken,* that is, if they appear collapsed because the essential humidity has been exhausted by the febrile heat, or if *the ears are cold and contracted:* coldness of the ears arising in an acute illness implies either absence of natural heat or an acute abscess arising internally, or absence of nutritive power. In the absence of natural heat, coldness of the ears results from the fact that heat first leaves those parts to which it returns last, and because it reaches the ears last, the ears become cold. They may become cold because of an acute abscess developing internally, for while the interior parts are suffering, and these are more noble than the exterior parts (**21**), the latter send their vigor and heat to the interior parts, and as a result the exterior parts, deprived of vigor and heat, become cold. Coldness of the ears may also imply a lack of nutritive power, because when an inadequate supply of nourishment is sent to the parts heat also does not arrive and nutrition suffers, whence the ears become cold. And being contracted because of contraction of the nerves, their fleshy parts become inverted because of deep corruption caused by a rise in heat which consumes the humidity.

If *the forehead is parched and drawn tight:* when such things occur in the exposed parts, what takes place within is much worse because of the greater degree of wasting, and *the color of the entire face becomes greenish,* indicating burning or mortification, *or pallid*, indicating the onset of mortification, or *lead-colored*, indicating profound destruction (**22**).

One should inquire about the appearance of the face at the beginning of the illness, that is, before beginning treatment, because the changes in features mentioned above may arise from poor health in general and not necessarily from a specific illness. If the changes do arise from poor health in general and not from a specific illness, or from lack of sleep, they are not to be feared. The body is weakened by lack of sleep and the changes mentioned above may occur, and therefore he says, one should *inquire whether the patient has long been sleepless or has had a persistent diarrhea. He inquires about diarrhea* because many of the above-mentioned symptoms may also develop from this cause; or *whether he has suffered from lack of food*, which may have the same effect. *If you find that any of these symptoms* did occur before the onset of the present illness, less danger is to be feared because such signs occur from impaired health in general and not necessarily from a specific disease. If they continue through the preceding night only they are not significant, *but if they continue for more than a day and a night*, then it is clear that the symptoms do proceed from the specific nature of the illness. *You shall not anticipate great danger if you recognize none of these symptoms* as arising from the disease itself, *but you may predict an early death* if these symptoms develop during the course of the disease, and develop directly from the nature of the disease itself.

In this manner an illness may go on for three days, that is, the harmful arrangement of signs may appear only after three days, if there has been a preceding diarrhea. *But there is still greater danger to be feared* because by this time, the diarrhea may have developed into a chronic condition. *You should inquire in detail about the body's previous appearance*, for not only must the signs mentioned above be inquired into, but also the body's appearance and especially the eyes (**23**). *For if they shun the light* this attempt to avoid glare indicates weakness of the spirit of vision which detaches itself from the atmosphere's brightness because of irritation and weakness. As a result, noticeable injury develops and thus the light flees. It may be said that in darkness, vision is suitable only for gathering objects together whereas in brightness, vision is suitable for separating objects. Every active agent in an illness takes on certain characteristics from the body in which it acts. Therefore, insane men tolerate suffering because the spirit of vision is great and strong or, if you prefer, because the organs of sight are very powerful (**24**). Nevertheless, if the sick do not tolerate suffering well and are not prepared to bear pain without worrying, then because the spirit of vision is weak and detaches itself quickly, and the organs of sight are also weak, tears fall involuntarily from the eyes. This signifies a strong reaction against the in-

trinsic humidity of the brain, which once in solution is emitted through the passages from which it drips down in the form of tears.

Or if the eyes protrude because of difficult breathing, or from choking caused by *humidity* filling the organs of respiration, then the breath imparts subtle bodies to the humors which rush to the eyes because they have a connection with them, thus causing them to protrude, or *if one seems smaller than the other*, this results from consumption of the essential humidity. Although either eye may be affected, it is usually the left because the accidental heat prevails much more strongly on the left side, whereas cold prevails just as strongly on the right.

And if the whites of the eyes are tinged with blood this indicates the presence of acute matter from which a stinging vapor (**25**) has been released; upon arriving at the eyes, it ruptures the vessels of the eyes, and thus blood escapes, resulting in redness. Also when there is a choking off of the breath, some breath, laden with blood, is sent with each respiration to the eyes and deposited there, causing the eyes to appear bloody. *At times the veins may seem black*, indicating mortification or inflammation, *or pallid*, indicating the onset of mortification. *If the eyes are turned upward and discharge freely*, this indicates the presence of strong heat acting deeply on the brain and destroying it, thus causing its humidity to descend to the eyes to be dried out by the exterior air and produce an ophthalmia (**26**). *If the eyes seem restless*: such instability may result from three causes—first, weakness or loss of the spirit of vision which, by detaching itself, produces an instability of the eyes; or from the presence of acute matter from which a pungent vapor is released which, arriving at the eyes stings and bites their tender substance, causing them to react to this danger by excessive mobility; or from severe dryness of the eyes which may result in mental alienation, followed by phrenitis. The consequent mental loss causes the eyes to move here and there and *to become tremulous*, indicating weakness of the regulating virtue of the eyes, and producing tremors such as are seen in paralytics. *Or they protrude excessively*: Hippocrates adds this for contrast to *those which are greatly sunken*, thus indicating the presence of strong heat consuming the substantial humidity of the eyes. This humidity being consumed, the eyes become smaller and therefore appear shrunken; or it may mean that the substantial heat of the nerves of the eye has been consumed by the strong heat, so that the nerves themselves are contracted, and these being contracted the eyes are retracted, or rather pulled upward, which indicates that a spasm will later result from inanition.

And the entire face appears livid, or greenish, which signifies definite changes in the entire constitution, and this must be considered a dangerous and often fatal sign.

It is necessary to examine the appearance of the eyes

even during sleep: the author has already prognosticated sufficiently about the disposition of the eyes when the patient is abnormally wakeful. Now he intends to prognosticate about their disposition during sleep, because from their disposition during sleep prognostic signs may be elicited concerning life or death. The eyelids are cartilaginous parts which cover the eyes and protect them from external injury. They have connections with the two membranes of the brain which protect that organ from external injury, namely the dura mater and the pia mater. From this it follows that when moist vapor derived from food and drink is dispersed and seeks the brain, which is—as it were—the furnace of the entire body, the vapor moistens and softens these membranes. Man is deprived of wakefulness through the moistening and relaxation of these membranes which have a connection with the eyelids, moisture producing relaxation and heaviness until the eyes are entirely covered.

It happens now and then that certain people have naturally large eyes and short eyelids, whereas others have shortened eyelids following diarrhea, so that in those who have naturally large eyes the whites may appear unusually prominent and this may also happen from diarrhea which causes a curvature of the eyelids. He implies that such signs are mortal because substantial humidity absorbed from food and drink was intended to moisten the membranes, namely the dura mater and the pia mater, and because these membranes and the eyelids have a common boundary the eyelids should likewise have been moistened and relaxed, but because the substantial humidity of the nerves coming to the eyelids was consumed by the action of febrile heat the nerves become contracted and the eyelids as well, so that the eyelids remain half-closed. And if the external parts are already consumed by heat the internal parts will soon become likewise involved, and this is what the author means.

And if only the whites can be seen through half-closed eyelids: the whites can be seen more readily than the black part, and we say this because when eyelids are half-closed they do not conceal the white of the eye, but the white and black appear to blend together. *If this does not result from diarrhea,* that is, if it does not occur from a spontaneous looseness of the bowels, *or from the operation of a cathartic,* that is, if it does not occur from the artificial action of medicine, *and if the patient does not normally sleep this way,* as those do who have large eyes and short eyelids, *then it is in fact a deadly symptom.* Because if this sign develops in a fresh state it will certainly happen in a dry one, and having occurred will lead to destruction. *And if the eyelids are contracted* from consumption of their innate humidity, thus making them appear turned upward, *or if the lower lids are likewise livid* because of mortification, *or if the nostrils are distorted* because of contraction of the nerves, *by these signs alone,* that is

unaccompanied, *or in association with those previously mentioned* you may judge that death is at hand.

4. [*Prognostics III*] *It is a good sign if the sick man, and so forth:* here the author prognosticates about the manner of reclining, because he says that from the patient's position in bed one may elicit indications of life or death. *It is good to find the patient reclining on either the right or left side* because when one lies comfortably and freely on either side, this eliminates the possibility of an abscess being present on both sides and additionally minimizes the danger of one developing on either side. Because an abscess is not present, there is less reason to anticipate choking or inflammation of the respiratory organs. When choking is not a factor, the patient is able to lie freely on either side, and when there is no inflammation of the respiratory organs, a man can draw air in freely to temper the innate heat and thus can lie safely on either side.

Although it is good to lie on either side, the question arises whether or not it is better to lie on the right side than on the left. We agree that it is better, having reasoned, *a priori,* that because the liver lies on the right side and is located under the stomach, the fire from this cauldron goes directly from the vicinity of the liver to the stomach, this being conducive to good digestion in the stomach and likewise in the liver. The resulting harmonious humidity induces an orderly and advantageous renewal of the spirits enabling the virtues to perform their functions more effectively. There is still another reason why it is better to lie on the right side than on the left, because catarrhal disease is more apt to become activated during sleep than during waking hours. During sleep, because of the activity of catarrhal disease, the natural heat is increased and this gives aid to the internal organs and their humors are dissolved (27). Being dissolved they reach the organs of breathing and the lungs, and because the lung is a concave, cavernous organ, humidity flowing into the lung can be retained without causing injury. Therefore the lung being on the right side it is better to lie on that side, whereas the heart, being located on the left side, has only a small concavity to retain the humidity without suffering injury.

With his hands, arms, legs and neck relaxed: the fact that the feet and hands are flexible indicates the sick man's ability to resist his illness. He adds, *not too flaccid,* but slightly rigid or firm; *and the entire body in a flexible position,* by which he implies ease of motion of the entire body. *The attitude of resting should* be the one which is customarily *adopted during health,* for it is desirable that sick persons settle themselves exactly as in health; and to lie in the position customary in health is best, even if he lies on the left side rather than the right, or even on his back.

For generally it is not a favorable sign to find the sick man lying on his back (28): this, only however, if it were not his usual practice, because such a position indicates a collection of pus developing on either side of the abdomen which causes him to lie this way, or it portends a sudden interference with breathing and inflammation of the organs of respiration, causing the supine person to seek fresh air. *If the arms and legs are extended and cold*, or not *equally warm, and if the patient suddenly slides from the head to the foot of the bed*, this implies mental alienation progressing to phrenitis (**29**), thus causing the man to act irrationally, twisting himself here and there; or when an inflammation of the breathing apparatus develops causing him to gasp for fresh air—this too may result in a movement from the head to the foot of the bed. *This is a most dangerous sign*, as we know from what has already been stated and from the mental involvement. *And if the legs are uncovered*, whether due to wasting of the flesh or from kicking off the bedclothes, the heat consumes the substantial humidity of the exposed lower members much more effectively than is the case with the upper limbs. *And if the legs are found slightly warm*, but not equally so, *and the neck is turned around with difficulty* through loss of the regulating virtue, *and if he thrashes his legs around*, these are very bad signs *indicating severe distress* from which the sick man's inability to sustain his illness can be inferred.

5. *If the sick man lies with his neck thrown back:* the author here lays down those signs derived from the appearance of the body which threaten sudden death, saying, *if the sick man lies with his neck thrown back*, his strength has become unequal to the task of sustaining the head. To the sick man his head has become a weight and a burden *and he lies with his mouth open:* this results either from exhaustion of the nerves leading to the jaw or from an attack of choking, so that he opens his mouth in order to draw in fresh air and thus avoid further choking, *and he lies with his feet twisted* because of contraction of the tendons going to the feet; for when the humidity concentrated in the tendons is consumed the tendons contract and the feet became twisted (**30**).

If lying on the abdomen is a position not customary in health (**31**): this implies either that the patient lies this way because of loss of consciousness and therefore does not know what he is doing; or he may lie this way because of some abscess developing in the abdomen, for when acute matter collects to form an abscess it induces pain, and the sufferer compresses his abdomen so that stupor and insensibility are induced and thus the pain is relieved, and hence this position indicates its cause. *For this is a bad sign and indicates delirium or pain* caused by an acute abscess arising within. *And if while in great distress he should suddenly try to pull himself erect*, this indicates a disturbance of the mind. *It is bad in every illness* for pus to flow freely because this indicates a rush of matter to the upper parts; but *it is worst in pneumonia*, for the lung, where pneumonia strikes, has free pas-

sages to the brain so that such matter ascends readily, seeks out the brain and accumulates to form a violent abscess (**32**).

6. *To grind the teeth in fevers and so forth:* the author now wishes to prognosticate about grinding of the teeth, a movement resulting from collision of one set of teeth with the other. Such grinding may be voluntary or involuntary: it is volunatry when done by the sick person either to terrify the bystanders or to move them to laughter, or it may arise when some pungent matter is dissolved into fumes through the action of heat. These fumes being very subtle are sent to the gums where they cause pain by stinging and biting. To avoid this pain the patient moves his teeth and hisses, and this leads to stupor and insensibility. If the grinding is involuntary it must come from depletion of the nerves leading to the lower jaw because when these nerves are contracted the lower jaw is contracted as well as the upper, and by such an alternating collision of the inferior molars with the superior the patient grinds his teeth. Such grinding of the teeth is bad because it indicates insanity and a rush of matter to the superior parts (**33**). Therefore he says, it is bad *to grind the teeth more than is usual*, that is, more than is customary among those who have a poor stomach and poor digestion, or who indiscreetly eat certain foods which produce an eructation because the stomach cannot retain them, with the result that the nerves leading to the lower jaw are replenished, causing a stridor of the teeth to occur. *But it is not harmful in children*, that is, in a child who is running a fever grinding of the teeth is not to be feared, because in children this occurs through an excess of humidity and the action of heat. When the heat is dispersed the nerves leading to the lower jaw are replenished, resulting in stridor of the teeth, and thus *grinding of the teeth portends death or madness* if it does not occur as a result of habit or in childhood.

7. *If an ulcer arises in the sick man's body:* the author intends to prognosticate about deadly abscesses arising during acute fevers from matter originating in the upper parts. Nature, debilitated by acute fevers, is not perfectly effective in a crisis and therefore does as well as it can, transmitting the harmful matter from the noble members to the ignoble. From this matter a hidden mass develops which is compressed to form an abscess, and such an abscess may arise during acute fevers from bile alone, or from blood alone. When derived from bile it is called "antrax" from "antrum," possibly because the place it occupies resembles a cave, or it is called "antrax" because it reflects the color of a cave. When the color is derived from blood it is called "carbuncle" from its resemblance to a live coal displaying a red color. An abscess derived from bile has a black color, for the dryness accentuates the heat which is seen at the edge, so that when ignited, it tends toward blackening, as may be seen in a blackened coal. When derived from blood,

an abscess exhibits a red color because the moisture of the blood, antagonizing the dryness, prevents the dryness from accentuating the heat, so that the red color persists.

But if one wishes to determine whether an abscess develops from the force of nature or from the force of disease, one must be attentive, for if the area occupied by the abscess does not diminish in size until after the evacuation of the noxious matter to the exterior, then it arises from the force of nature. If the abscess becomes concealed the area which it abandons must still be watched, for if a color develops there from a humor coursing around, this is a good sign, and occurs through natural powers, but when the natural heat is strengthened, all the harmful matter is destroyed so that the color of a harmful humor ought not to appear. But if there remains a trace of the harmful humor, it must originate from an unnatural force, and this evil matter either sends off satellites or itself becomes so rarified that it travels to one of the principal parts and thus induces death, and this is what he says.

Then he adds: *if an ulcer appears on the sick man's body* during convalescence it is not to be feared, but one should note *whether the carbuncle developed before or during the illness*, because either may occasionally happen. It is quite important to decide whether the ulcer appeared after the onset of the illness, because a dried, concealed greenish ulcer indicates the presence of an unnatural force; a *yellowish color* indicates the presence of bile, while a leaden gray color indicates mortification and *signifies impending death* from the rush of harmful matter to the brain resulting in disruption of its substance and a fatal ending.

8. [*Prognostics IV*] *Note these signs about the movement of the hands:* Hippocrates now undertakes to make certain predictions from a study of the movements of the hands in acute fevers and in peripneumonic abscesses because from such a study some indication may be drawn concerning the likelihood of recovery or death. *In acute fevers such as in pneumonia* the harmful matter is diverted to the superior parts and heat which dissolves the matter aids this process, with the result that the patient moves his hands about as if trying to assemble something. This results from acute matter stinging and biting the tender and noble substance of the face, so that he throws his hands to his face. Such movements of the hands occur in pneumonia because the lungs have free passages to the superior parts, and as the matter travels about the patient places his hands on his face because of the fury of the matter. *Also in a false phrenitis:* a false phrenitis is said to occur from humors inactivating the spirit of vision. *And with severe pain of the head they also raise their hands to the face* because of the rush of matter to the upper parts *moving them here and there* in an attempt to escape the biting and stinging. The patient touches his hands to his face

as though he had placed something there or *as though he were collecting or searching for something*, all of which implies a dissemination of the harmful matter; or *he may pick something off his clothes* because certain subtle vapors which inactivate the spirit of vision irritate him as would imaginary flies or even blades of grass. *If he is seen to pick at the walls this is a bad and mortal sign*, a warning of impending madness (**34**).

9. [*Prognostics V*] *If breathing is hurried and so forth:* the author now intends to draw some indications from the action of inspiration (**35**), for *when the breathing is hurried*, inspired air is repeatedly taken in by the action of inspiration and expiration, being received as inhaled air and emitted as exhaled air; but if the air exhaled through the nose and mouth is cold, this is a fatal sign. Inhalation results from the action of a certain airy substance which arouses the physical and other virtues, as has been stated here. The air is taken in by the process of inspiration and expiration, but such action may be deep or shallow, frequent or infrequent. Deep breathing arises from heat, shallow from cold, infrequent from humidity, frequent from dryness. Deep breathing arises from heat in this manner: when the organs of respiration are disturbed by an excess of heat, the heart, because of this excessive heat, desires to draw in more cold air, but more air cannot be drawn in unless the heart is dilated, and deep inspiration follows such a great dilatation, but because there is great dilatation, there is also great contraction which results in deepened respiration. Or, to put it in another way, heat brings about the generation of vapors, and because of this heat the many dissolved vapors which have centripetal motion bring about a great dilatation, and because an excess of these vapors is capable of extinguishing the heart's heat a strong contraction results in order to effect the emission of superfluous vapors.

Cold results in shallow inspiration and expiration, for when the organs of respiration are in disorder cold does not permit the generation of vapors. Therefore more air is inhaled in order to reduce the heart's heat, but less air results in less dilatation, and thus if the inspiration is shallow the dilatation will be small, the contraction will also be small and the resulting respiration shallow. Or because cold has a strong motion to the center it always results in a shallow inspiration and expiration.

Dryness produces rapid respiration because dryness being the refinement of heat (**36**) aggravates it and strong heat results in a great dilatation. But because dryness also has a motion to the center tending toward contraction, it prevents this great dilatation from taking place, so that what is required in quantity is supplied by periodic interchange. Very infrequent respiration occurs through humidity; such humidity by dulling the heat of the heart results in rarified breathing. Therefore he says *if respiration is fre-*

quent, that is, if inspiration and expiration are hurried, *and there is sign of pain*, that is, of the matter which induces pain, *and of excessive heat*, by which the organs of respiration become inflamed, then as a result of this pain there develops a frequency of inspiration and expiration, because all pain aggravates the catarrhal circulation and the humors run down to the painful area, and from such an excess of humors there develops a narrowing of the passages. From such narrowing and from the excessive flow of humors the heart becomes accelerated with resulting frequency of inspiration and expiration.

If in those organs which lie above the diaphragm: the ancient physicians (**37**) who scrutinized the interior of the human body found the organs of respiration lying above the diaphragm, a thick membrane which separates the organs of respiration from the organs of digestion. *And if the breathing is deep*, that is, if there is deep inspiration and expiration *with some interruption*, that is, if with the shortness of breath there is also a forceful expulsion of air, then from such forced expiration the living being becomes oblivious of his normal actions and loses consciousness, *and alienation of the spirit results*, for rapid inspiration with interruption portends alienation, and such rapid inspiration may arise from a multitude of causes. Intermittency of respiration implies a rise of matter to the upper parts, with resulting alienation (**38**). *And if indeed cold air is exhaled through the nose and mouth this is a mortal sign*, for such simple continuous relaxation of the breath must be differentiated from the normal act of inspiration and expiration, and quite simply the inhalation of cold air, *and its exhalation is a mortal sign* because it signifies extinction of the natural heat in the heart, and hence death. In fact, death is nothing more than the extinction of the natural heat in the heart.

An easy respiration, that is, an easy action of inspiration and expiration *and a regular rhythm* are to be hoped for, because respiration which is neither too frequent nor too deep is a sure sign indicating health. *During acute illnesses accompanied by fever* if the action of inspiration and expiration is orderly, then there is also an orderly disposition of the heart—the organ which is necessary for life—and of the parts adjacent to the heart.

10. [*Prognostics VI*] *A good and favorable sweat and so forth:* as we have stated above every sign is derived either from the form of the body, from its superfluities or from its actions. The author has already spoken at sufficient length about signs which arise from the body's form; now he plans to discuss signs which arise from superfluities.

It should be noted that there are four discharges from the body, namely sputum, feces, urine, and sweat, and depending on the diseased part of the body from which it arises, each discharge has its special significance. Sputum reveals the state of the animate members, that is, of the respiratory organs and the stomach, while the fecal discharge indicates abnormalities of the alimentary tract, including the stomach and intestines. Urine reveals the state of the liver and urinary organs; sweat, by inference, the disposition of the entire body.

Sweat is a humid vapor excreted from the body through the pores, thus moistening the skin (**39**). It is variously considered as to quantity, quality, lightness or heaviness, duration, and location. The quantity may be large or small, and the quantity may result from either natural or unnatural causes. A heavy sweat occurs naturally when nature eliminates well-digested and well-dissolved matter through the usual channels, with the result that the sick man feels easier and more comfortable, and indeed is restored to health. A heavy sweat may also occur through unnatural forces when certain members are incapable of resisting the pressure of excessive matter, and because these parts cannot resist the humors there is an excessive discharge of humors, including not only those which are superfluous but also those which are beneficial. A mild scanty sweat occurs naturally when nature removes harmful matter through other channels than the pores, so that little matter remains in the abdomen; such a sweat is light and watery. A light sweat may also occur through unnatural forces when there is weakness of the expulsive power.

Sweat is considered as to quality in several ways, namely as to color, odor, and taste: if it is clear in color this indicates an excess of natural phlegm; if red, an abundance of blood; if saffron-colored, of bile; if lead-colored, of black bile. As to odor: it is thought that a fetid odor indicates a serious corruption of the parts; as to taste: it is thought that lack of taste indicates an excess of natural phlegm; a sweet taste, an excess of blood or sweet phlegm; a vinegary taste, an excess of black bile or sour phlegm; a bitter taste, an excess of bile (**40**). With regard to lightness: it is thought that a watery sweat indicates an abundance of the more subtle and lighter humors, whereas if the sweat becomes thickened and almost solid this indicates an excess of the solid and thick humors. In regard to quality, sweat may also be considered in another way, that is, with respect to warmth and coldness, because warm sweat implies a lesser illness, cold a more serious one. As to time: it is thought that sweating should occur on the critical day appointed by nature for this task, because through such an elimination the patient is made to feel easier and more comfortable. As to location: it is thought that sweating should occur uniformly throughout the body, thus indicating a general discharge of the harmful humors, for if sweating does not occur uniformly throughout the body, then the location of the sweat is related to the site of the illness, and a cold sweat of the head and neck is a dangerous sign, indicating a serious loss of natural heat.

A good and laudable sweat is one which appears on the critical day in all acute illnesses, that is, it occurs on the day appointed for this task, and *relieves the patient* by eliminating harmful humors throughout every possible channel. *And that sweat is desirable* which appears uniformly throughout the body, because this indicates the strength of the expulsive power, and *by such a sweat the patient is made to feel easier and more comfortable*. The body is weakened by the presence of an aggravating humor, whereas by its elimination the patient is made easier and more comfortable. *But if the sweats do not produce these effects they are useless*, and if they do not occur on a critical day they will fail to relieve the sick man. And if the sweat does not appear uniformly over the body, and the sick man is not made easier or more comfortable, then indeed his condition may be aggravated through retention of the humor and his body may be weakened. *But a cold sweat is harmful* because it indicates extinction of natural heat or the presence of cold matter which requires a long period for digestion, so that before it can be digested the patient becomes enfeebled while the disease becomes ever more powerful in the fight against nature. *Cold sweat confined to the head and neck is dangerous* because coldness develops from extinction of natural heat in the head and passes through the neck into the heart. Hippocrates refers especially to these parts in which the attractive force is so powerful that when humors are dissolved they pass into sweat, and in certain acute fevers this may forecast death through extinction of natural heat. *And if the sweat is of long duration*, this indicates the elimination of much matter by the patient and this is a good sign.

[*Prognostics VII*] It is best *if the hypochondria are free of pain*: the author plans to make prognostications based on the condition of the hypochondria. These are concave regions containing free space and lying underneath the soft parts of the ribs. (41). It is known that there are four hypochondria—two superior lying above the diaphragm and two inferior below the diaphragm. The right superior hypochondrium has the largest cavity and this is filled almost entirely by the lung; the left superior hypochondrium has a smaller cavity which contains the heart; the left inferior hypochondrium also has a large cavity filled by the spleen; the right inferior hypochondrium is filled in large part by the liver.

Whenever an unnatural humor develops this is confined (42) within the hypochondria, and the resulting excessive heat leads to crust formation and an abscess. Therefore it is good to find the hypochondria free of pain, because when there is no pain we know that there is no circulation of the humors, and just as a circulation of the humors may lead to the formation of an abscess so does the absence of the humors preclude the possibility of an abscess. Because the hypochondria are free of pain this indicates

that the phlegmatic humor which causes diffuse pain and the bilious humor which causes a stabbing pain are not present in great strength, and this is plain. And if the hypochondria are soft, this indicates that the dryness which destroys humidity does not predominate so that a natural softness pervades the hypochondria.

If the hypochondria are in good order on both sides the outlook is favorable, that is, if both upper and lower hypochondria have the conformation normally expected, *this is a good sign* because it indicates that they are not being irritated by any specific humor, and that no specific humor has gathered there to be collected into an abscess.

But if there is fever or pain the cause may be the descent of the sanguine humor with resulting abscess formation, *or if there is spasm and distension* the cause may be the presence of phlegmatic matter which fills the hypochondria and spreads laterally. *The hypochondria may differ in appearance* depending on whether there is an accumulation of phlegm or black bile and whether only one or both hypochondria are involved. It is therefore important to determine whether the matter which has collected to form an abscess is derived from bile or blood, for *if a pulsation or bounding exists in any part of the hypochondria* this indicates that the matter is composed of bile which has been dispersed and dissolved, and once dissolved has sought an exit, but being unable to find one because of the crust it has broken through the crust and thus has produced a pulsation. *This implies severe distress and delirium:* severe distress arises from the presence of the sanguine humor which produces choking, while delirium arises from the presence of black bile, because bilious matter, becoming easily refined and dissolved, seeks the upper parts and eventually produces delirium, so that *in this particular condition* disease has its origin at the very point where the humors have accumulated.

11. *The eyes should be examined* because matter passes through them, and if they move about rapidly this is due to a stinging and biting which causes the eyes to move rapidly in reaction to this irritation. This unfavorable sign indicates the abduction of matter to the upper parts resulting in corruption of the anterior cell of the head.

If a gathering develops during the course of an acute illness this indicates that the fever has already done as much harm as possible. *If there is pain and swelling in the hypochondria so that both hpyochondria are tense this is a very bad sign* because even a single abscess in one hypochondrium is sufficient to cause destruction; *but if only one hypochondrium is involved* it is better to find the left side involved rather than the right, in other words, this is less harmful, especially if the upper left hypochondrium has been spared and only the left lower hypochondrium is involved, because this contains the spleen which is an ignoble member (43). But if the gathering develops in the left superior hypochondrium this is a very bad sign because there lies the heart, the part appointed to protect life (44).

If a gathering begins at the onset of the disease it may not cause death immediately, and if it lasts until the twentieth day and neither pain nor fever diminish, then because of the continued involvement of the part *the gathering is converted into an abscess* by the persistent action of heat, and the matter having come to a boil is then converted into sanies. *Often in these cases there is a useful flow of blood from the nostrils within a period of seven days:* this demonstrates the very great strength of nature in opening new channels distinct from the usual passages, and there is nothing more beneficial. *One should inquire about pain in the forehead*, for when the matter of an abscess needs to be drained off there is pain in the forehead because some of the matter has risen to the superior parts, and such signs are of prognostic value. *One should also inquire about dimness of vision* caused by matter rising to the superior parts. *You may anticipate a nosebleed* because of ruptured venules, *especially in those who are less than thirty-five* and have an excess of bilious humor.

12. *But if a soft swelling and so forth:* the author plans at this point to make certain predictions based on the variety of abscesses, the humors which produce them, and variations in time of development and location. Some abscesses are derived from blood, others from bile and still others from phlegm or black bile. Our author intends first to discuss abscesses derived from sanguine humor, but concerning this variety we note a difference of opinion, for Johannitius claims that the sanguine abscess is firm while Hippocrates asserts that it is soft and movable to touch, adding that blood may be natural or unnatural, the natural being found in the arteries and veins (45). Because blood when present within the vessels shares in a measure of firmness, the abscess formed from this blood is also firm, and it is to this type that Johannitius is referring. On the other hand Hippocrates is considering abscesses composed of unnatural blood, or ichor, so that when he says *if a soft abscess develops*, he means that this type results from watery matter which modifies the essential nature of the sanguine abscess so that it becomes soft *and painless* or, more accurately, without severe pain. All this implies the presence of cold matter because cold makes the part resistant and insensitive to pain, so that we call such minimal pain, "painless," that is, it is free from destructive and harmful qualities; *and movable to touch*, not that it ought to be touched, but if accessible it will yield readily to the slightest pressure owing to softness, leaving a deep hole because the essential nature of the matter has been so greatly modified by humidity. *Very often the condition will resolve itself as already indicated*, that is, by a severe nosebleed, or by the blood being changed into sanies, or in the manner already described by Hippocrates as typical of younger patients.

But if it lasts until the sixtieth day: this lemma does not apply to the preceding variety of abscess, but to one formed of black bile and, like all general statements, it does not necessarily apply to each individual case, *and fever is present*, because fever is often associated with a slowly developing abscess, *then the matter is changed into pus*, that is, the matter having come to a boil by the persistence of heat, is converted into sanies.

And every abdominal abscess can be judged by this rule, namely, that it will terminate either by conversion into sanies or by a strong discharge of blood. *But a solid abscess:* here he intends to discuss an abscess formed of bile which he calls "firm," because the matter collected to form such an abscess is warm and dry. And even though heat acts to bring about resolution, dryness acts to produce wasting so that the end result is firmness of the abscess, *with pain*, and such severe pain arising from these destructive and harmful qualities *is to be* feared and mistrusted because it implies the presence of very acute and violent matter *which is swiftly fatal* and which can kill by its own virulence through the destruction of some principal member, and therefore *is to be feared* and mistrusted as is any terrible danger.

But those abscesses which are soft: having discussed the bloody and bilious abscesses, our author now intends to discuss the phlegmatic abscess. We are already familiar with the signs of the bloody and bilious abscess, and because he now describes the phlegmatic abscess as *soft and painless* he seems to be repeating here what he has already said about the bloody abscess being soft and movable to the touch, but in fact he states that the phlegmatic abscess becomes *fluctuating to touch*, and it should be noted that there is a distinction between "movable" and "fluctuating," the latter implying a sort of running here and there, and the idea of greater mobility than is implied in the term "movable to touch." *And these* abscesses *are soft* because humidity produces a softening of matter, *and painless*, because an excess of cold induces lack of sensibility so that pain is not felt. *The phlegmatic abscess is resolved more slowly than the one derived from bile*, so that death approaches more gradually.

But an abscess in the region of the abdomen: the author now prognosticates about the quantiy of matter which may collect in various parts of the body, noting that at different locations the quantity of matter may vary from time to time. *An abscess in the region of the abdomen* accumulates less of the humors, because the abdomen does not contain much free space and there are many channels of elimination, whereas the hypochondria not only contain larger free cavities but have no channels of elimination so that a greater quantity of matter tends to accumulate in the hypochondria. *Least harmful of all abscesses are those which develop below the umbilicus* because the umbilicus and channels of elimination occupy a great part of the free space in this cavity. *A sign much to be hoped for* is an effusion of blood, because this indicates nature's ability to discover new channels for the elimination of matter *from those abscesses found in the above mentioned places*, that is, for eliminating the sanies found there. Hippocrates implies that it is better to eliminate blood already changed into sanies than blood which has not gone through this process, because sanies does not corrupt the part in which it develops.

13. *Every long-lasting abscess:* now he prognosticates about the abscess formed of black bile, characterizing this type as long-lasting either because of a special virtue or excellence or because it is derived from solid, cold, and dry matter and therefore usually terminates after a much longer period than any other abscess, possibly within sixty days. *Every long-lasting abscess in the places previously mentioned will eventually be converted into pus*, so that it is necessary to observe carefully, and so forth: the master then introduces three useful considerations about abscesses, relating to form, time of rupture, and conversion of the contents into sanies.

First, he considers the form of the abscess, and whether this be favorable or unfavorable, for indeed if the abscess projects to a point this means that the matter is gathering to the outside and is not incorporated in the flesh and is, in fact, distinct from it. Therefore the flesh itself is not affected, but as a result of great strength of the natural heat a movement of matter develops from the sides to the center, thus forming a point. This form is good and the rupture of such an abscess is favorable for the matter is expelled outwardly and not internally; but if it breaks internally the part becomes purulent on the surface and the medication applied cannot successfully bring about its effect without losing strength. If indeed the abscess ruptures externally this is desirable because the matter not being incorporated in the flesh does not cause the flesh to become infected and the medication may operate more effectively.

The formation of pus which is white in color is laudable, because it indicates that the matter is not raw but well-digested and homogeneous throughout and free from an evil odor, and this is what he says (**46**).

14. *Therefore it is necessary to watch closely those abscesses which are developing pus*, that is, are becoming softened before rupturing. *Following this rule* we agree that in those abscesses *which swell slightly but do not break externally* the matter becomes incorporated in the flesh, and *spreads internally to a small degree*; but since there is little of such an abscess below the surface we must clearly be suspicious of the presence of another hidden more deeply within. *And the very pointed abscess is favorable*, this form being attributed to the strength of the heat which produces a movement of matter from the sides to the center, thus forming

a point. If the abscess does not project to a point this implies a weakness of the heat which may lead to gangrene.

Those abscesses which are broad: this form occurs when matter, becoming incorporated in the flesh, putrifies and destroys it, and *the least pointed are very bad* because they indicate weakness of natural heat and inability of matter to follow its proper movement, that is, from the sides to the center, where it should project into a point; and if the heat is weak this implies the extinction of nature. *Those abscesses which rupture internally but also have an external outlet are worst:* this means that if the abscess ruptures internally and externally it must extend in both directions, and this happens only when an excess of humor is concentrated within the abscess which, by its presence, breaks through the inner part as well as the outer. *If there is no communication to the exterior this is better:* it has been correctly stated that when matter is collected to the outside and there is evidence of softening this is a good sign. He also means that when an *internal abscess has no external outlet this is not a bad but a good sign* (**47**).

And that pus which is white is laudable for by the continued power of heat matter is converted into pus *which is uniform throughout*, and has not been left uneven through weakness of the heat; *and this pus is also uniform at the surface* because there is an absence of flatulence *and bad odor*, either fetid or heavy; a fetid odor indicates corruption of the humors, a heavy odor corruption of the parts. *Pus which is colored other than white is much worse* because just as laudable pus is praiseworthy so must harmful pus be condemned because it indicates corruption of the humors and of the parts.

SECTION TWO

15. [*Prognostics VIII*] *All dropsies and so forth:* this is the beginning of the second part which is devoted to a study of the natural virtue, and the signs considered here are all related to the strength or weakness of the natural virtue. This part begins with a study of dropsy which usually has its origin in a defect of the digestive virtue of the liver. We must therefore study just what dropsy is, how many forms it may take, from what causes it may arise, which of these forms are curable and which incurable, and why they are curable or incurable.

Dropsy is described by Galen in the *Passionarius* as a defect of the digestive virtue of the liver, and by Constantinus in the *Viaticum* as an aberration of the digestive virtue of the liver (**48**). These definitions refer to the cause, for dropsy is not a defect by itself, but arises from a defect of the digestive virtue of the liver (**49**). Dropsy is a swelling or unnatural enlargement of the parts which arises from a dysfunction of the digestive virtue of the liver. When Hippocrates speaks of swelling he refers to two varieties, namely, white swelling and anasarca or hyposarca. The warm humor must be present in these cases because heat is very effective in producing such swellings. When he speaks about enlargements with bloating he refers to two other varieties, namely, tympanites and ascites. Thus, there are four varieties of dropsy: white swelling, anasarca or hyposarca, tympanites and ascites. White swelling is so called from "leucoë" which means "white," and "flegmantia" meaning "phlegm," because this variety of dropsy is composed of white or so-called natural phlegm. Hyposarca is so called from "ypos" which means "under," and "sarcos" which means "flesh" because in this variety of dropsy the matter is localized underneath the flesh. Anasarca is so called from "ana" which means "close to" and "sarcos," "flesh," because in this variety, the matter is located adjacent to the flesh. Tympanites is so called from "tympanum" or "drum," because the abdomen of these patients, when struck, resounds like a drum. Ascites is so called from the word "ἀσκος" or "venter" because the abdomen of such persons has the consistency of a half-filled wine-skin (50).

White swelling arises from a universal dysfunction of the liver when cold and humidity are present in almost equal strength; anasarca is produced by a universal dysfunction of the liver when cold and dryness are present in almost equal strength. Tympanities arises from a dysfunction of the liver when heat and dryness are present in almost equal strength in the convexity, while cold predominates in the concavity. Ascites may arise from a dysfunction of the liver when heat and humidity are present in almost equal strength in the convexity while cold predominates in the concavity. But it should be noted that such a universal dysfunction of the liver produced by cold and humidity results in an impairment of digestion, and this impairment of digestion by cold and humidity leads in turn to the generation of an excess of phlegmatic humor, the cold causing constriction while the humidity causes softening, thus increasing the strength of the expulsive virtue. Then the phlegmatic humor thus engendered is carried by vessels throughout the entire body, giving rise to a certain type of dropsy which is called white swelling.

A universal dysfunction of the liver produced by cold and dryness in almost equal strength results in an impairment of digestion and it is this impairment of digestion produced by constricting cold and destructive dryness which leads to the generation of an excess of superfluities. The constriction caused by cold strengthens the expulsive virtue which in the presence of destructive dryness acts on the superfluities to produce flatulence, so that the generation of superfluities depends on the strength of the expulsive virtue, and as a result of the pressure of the flatulence on the superfluities a swelling is produced. The flatulence being heavy seeks an exit, but being unable to find one becomes crushed and corrupted, and this leads

to fetor. This type of swelling is called hyposarca or anasarca.

Likewise, when a dysfunction of the convexity of the liver develops through heat and dryness the pores are opened by the relaxing quality of the heat so that spirits and humors are expelled. Asthma develops from such opened pores because of cold which predominates in the concavity. This cold impairs digestion and leads to the excessive production of superfluities, and because these are disintegrated by heat and destructive dryness there results an enormous generation of wind. This wind, being trapped between the convexity of the liver and the peritoneum, cannot leave because of the liver's attractive power so that the wind inflates the entire abdomen, and this type is called tympanites. Again, when a dysfunction of the convexity develops through heat and humidity, the pores are opened by this heat and the spirits and humors are expelled through the open pores, thus causing asthma. The coldness in the concavity and the humidity result in a great generation of superfluities which, being acted upon by the heat of the convexity, terminate in watery discharges. And the heat which disintegrates the superfluities results in a generation of wind which accumulates between the omentum and the peritoneum, thus causing the swelling known as ascites.

Having devoted enough attention to the varieties of dropsy we must now look to the causes from which dropsy develops. Dropsy is an aberration of function arising principally from the liver, but it may also arise from a disorder of the intestines, stomach, organs of respiration, spleen, and the kidneys, as well as from an excessive loss or retention of blood. As we have seen earlier dropsy arises most often from a defect of the liver or, to put it somewhat differently, the defect of the liver arises from an abscess forming within the liver which weakens it so severely that the liver cannot digest the ptisane sent to it. Thus all digestion is impaired and in this manner dropsy arising from a defect of the stomach has its origin, for the function of any organ is prefixed and predetermined so that it performs its duty properly and no other organ can perform it. Thus it becomes impossible for the third digestion to be effective in the various organs, if digestion in the stomach is impaired, because the liver cannot substitute for the stomach, so that when digestion in the stomach is impaired digestion of the liver is also impaired and thus a dropsy develops.

Dropsy may also arise from disorders of the intestine, from retention of fecal material in constipation or from severe diarrhea. In cases of constipation, when feces cannot be eliminated, the ptisane drawn to the liver becomes mixed with fecal material and corrupted; as a result heat is lost, digestion is impeded, and this impairment of digestion leads to dropsy. In cases of severe diarrhea the ptisane is sent directly to the intestines and passes out through them without being first sent to the liver to rekindle the liver's natural heat. Because the humidity in cereal foods helps to maintain heat, when this humidity is absent heat conceals itself and the opposite quality, namely cold, makes an appearance; through cold, digestion is impaired, and this impairment of digestion leads to dropsy.

Dropsy may also occur in cases of disorder of the breathing apparatus, because when the organs of respiration are disordered by excessive heat and dryness a thirst develops in the stomach with dryness at the orifice so that the patient imbibes an excessive quantity of water. This water impedes the first digestion, and, if the first digestion is impaired, so will be the second, with the result that dropsy develops. Or dropsy develops because the attractive virtue which abounds when heat and dryness predominate in the organs of respiration passes through a branch of the vena cava (51) with the result that the vena cava drains the unpurified secretion of the liver from the smaller veins so that digestion is impaired, and this impairment of digestion leads to dropsy.

Dropsy may arise from a disorder of the spleen, because when this organ is obstructed and swollen it presses on the liver; also when the spleen is obstructed it cannot receive the black bile which acts in the spleen as a purifying agent. Because this black bile remains in the liver it weakens the liver by its coldness and both qualities combine to interfere with digestion so that an impairment of digestion results which leads to dropsy (52). Also when the liver is compressed by the swollen spleen ptisane cannot be digested, indigestion results and then dropsy. Dropsy may arise from a disorder of the kidneys when, as in diabetes, the attractive virtue thrives in the kidneys, thus drawing uncocted juice to these organs, the heat is diminished and the contrary quality, namely cold, becomes strengthened, thus producing an impairment of digestion and dropsy. A dropsy may occur from an excessive loss of blood, because blood is the nourishment of heat, so that when blood and heat are lacking there is an interference with digestion in the stomach, and dropsy results. Or from retention of blood, for when blood is retained and becomes redundant in the liver it weakens the liver, thus producing an impairment of digestion and dropsy.

We must now consider which forms of dropsy are curable and which are incurable, or rather difficult to cure: those curable are white swelling and anasarca or hyposarca; tympanites and ascites are difficult to cure. White swelling and anasarca or hyposarca are properly considered curable because they arise from a general dysfunction of the liver, white swelling from a natural dysfunction through cold and humidity, anasarca from a general dysfunction through cold and dryness. Because contraries are cured by contraries, contraries antagonistic to each morbid condition can

be administered in the form of the contrary quality, thus leading the body back to health. Just as heat and dryness are antagonistic to white swelling, so are cold and humidity antagonistic to anasarca or hyposarca. In another way these conditions may be considered curable because the medication taken in by the body is aided by the virtues, and because the expulsive virtue is strong in both conditions the medication assists in the removal of the harmful humors from which dropsy originates. There is still another explanation, namely that these two forms of dropsy originate from a humor, and since the medication binds itself to the humor and follows it into the solid tissue to which the humor belongs both are removed and the illness terminates. On the other hand, the two remaining forms are difficult to cure because the qualities in both are antagonistic and disordered.

Tympanites arises from a dysfunction of the convexity of the liver through heat and dryness, while the concavity remains cold; in these cases warm things cannot be administered because of the dysfunction of the convexity through heat, for every like augments its like and may produce an exacerbation of the dysfunction, and, because the concavity is cold, cold things cannot be administered. Lukewarm things should be administered least of all because everything which is less harmful becomes altered by contact with more harmful, and so on. Again, medications which are carried by the expulsive virtue are not useful because these dropsies arise from a defect of the expulsive virtue. Furthermore these forms of dropsy have an excess of flatulence so that the medication cannot find an attachment to the matter which is light and delicate. Thus the flatulence cannot be expelled, and in fact medication may produce a greater generation of flatulence and thus aggravate the problem.

16. *All dropsies arising in acute illnesses:* it would seem contrary to nature for dropsy to occur during an acute illness with fever because such a disease is warm and accidental heat is present, whereas dropsy was called a cold disease in the explanation. Although dropsy is a cold disease in potentiality fever is a warm disease in actuality and a warm disease in actuality is not antagonistic to one which is cold in potentiality. *Every dropsy arising in acute diseases is harmful* because fever is a warm disease and dropsy is a cold disease. Warm medications cannot be usefully prescribed for fever or cold things for dropsy and lukewarm things are least useful. *Indeed dropsy is aggravated by fever, head colds, and pain.* By this comment the author wishes to indicate that it is bad when dropsy is accompanied by fever because fever is so much like this disease that the nature of both is altered. It is also bad if dropsy comes on with a head cold because this indicates repletion, and the head cold is evidently a subordinate condition arising through a defect of form, and when this subordinate

character is modified, the humor causing repletion spreads widely, causing a solution of continuity. If pain accompanies the dropsy this is also a bad sign because the character of the disease has been modified in various ways and even a nature formed of all the virtues cannot withstand the disease (53), whether this be of a similar nature, a subordinate nature or a combination of both.

Dropsy with fever is bad and usually arises from the lumbar and iliac regions: the author intends to indicate where dropsy has its origin, and shows that it may develop in the loins or kidneys, for certainly the kidneys when completely desiccated by thirst, as in diabetes, draw in the uncocted juice of ptisane, thus impeding the second digestion, and the resulting indigestion leads to dropsy through this defect of the kidneys. "Ilia" are called intestines by substituting a part for the whole, and dropsy may result from constipation or diarrhea, as has already been said, or may occasionally appear from a malfunction of the small intestine when wind is imprisoned there and colic develops. In such intestines the superfluous matter of the first digestion is diverted to the liver where it adulterates the juice of the ptisane which in turn impairs the second digestion and thus dropsy develops.

Some cases arise from the liver: that is, one variety arises from a general defect of the liver, others arise from a natural dysfunction of the liver through cold and humidity or cold and dryness, while still others arise from a defect of the convexity through heat and humidity when cold of almost equal strength is present in the concavity. Or dropsy may arise from an abscess *originating in the lumbar region,* that is, in the kidneys, or from the ilia or intestines, *as becomes evident from a swelling of the feet.* For when dropsy arises from a dysfunction of the intestines as a result of constipation an immoderate amount of superfluous matter is attracted to the liver, thus causing the liver to be weakened, with the result that the accidental heat from the impaired digestion generates a heavy wind whose thick fumes are sent thouogh all branches of the chylous vein to the lower parts by the saphenous veins, thus causing the feet to become swollen. *Or dropsy may arise from a protracted diarrhea* when the dropsy is complicated by an excessive abdominal discharge or by an elimination through the channel of the penis. The abdomen has two ways of cleansing itself, one through the pudic circle, the other through the penis. This elimination occurs through the penis because the kidneys which were desiccated, having drawn up a great quantity of juices, expel much of these through the penis. *Nor in fact is there much relief of pain,* for the discomfort is not derived from the humor but from the spreading of the excess flatulence, *or of abdominal swelling* because the excessive abdominal flatulence joins with the humor in forming this swelling *which originates in the liver* or rather from a defect of the liver.

A non-productive cough results whose cause is ultimately a defect of the liver, and this slight cough may originate from a general dysfunction of the liver or from a dysfunction of the convexity or from an abscess (54). For when there is a great accumulation of humors in the liver this organ becomes swollen and presses on the stomach, and the stomach compresses the organs of respiration which in turn compress the trachea, thus causing an irritation of the airway and a cough. *But there is no expectoration* because there is no matter in the organs of respiration, *and the feet swell* because of the excess flatulence sent down to the feet through the third branch of the chylous vein, *but they eliminate only a small quantity* because the expulsive virtue fails. Feces are retained and constipation occurs with tympanites, *and all this with distress* because the stool is small and hard *and abscesses which develop in the abdominal region* have their origin in the superfluities generated by such impaired digestion. But there are also false swellings resembling abscesses produced by imprisoned flatulence *which cannot immediately reach the outside* because the fumes are too heavy to be expelled daily through the pores (55), and *this flatulence moves about from place to place* because the fumes have no fixed location.

[Prognostics IX] *If the head, palms and soles are cold:* in an acute fever with severe dropsy coldness of the extremities is a bad sign, for this condition may arise from a failure of natural heat or from a lack of nutrition. And just as impaired digestion results in a lack of nutrition, so does lack of food result in a loss of heat because humor is the nutrient of nature as food is of the body. All this becomes understandable with some effort.

And if the abdomen, flanks and jaws are warm this is also a bad sign because it is through an impairment of digestion that the accidental heat rises and warms the abdomen, and through their common boundary, the jaws as well. *It is best if the entire body is of uniform temperature* because then there is no loss of natural heat or lack of nutrition *and the patient is easy and turns freely* and the skin shows no roughness because irritating dryness is absent, and such natural softness is good because it indicates the absence of dryness which consumes the humidity. *It is good if the patient can move about easily and quickly* because the irritating humor from the superfluities is absent, and because this aggravating humor is not present the patient appears more comfortable. *But if he is difficult to move* because of the irritating humors or because there is a lack of spirit *and the hands and feet are heavy* because of the aggravating humor and lack of spirit, then the governing virtue is incapable of sustaining the parts in their proper order and position, and such signs *are ominous* of impending death.

If indeed lividity is observed arising from cold which results in an impairment of digestion this occurs because the cold producing this impairment of digestion causes an aqueous fluid to be expressed from the indigestable matter, just as may be seen in a winepress when the residue settles to the bottom, and this indigestible matter causes the fingertips to be stained a leaden color.

But if the fingernails are greenish in color this color is attributed to matter generated by destructive cold combined with a substance generated by burning heat, and *death may soon be expected* because the cold and hot matter present are both excessive, and through the hot matter there results an inflammation of the heart, the organ entrusted with life. *If a leaden color predominates,* this indicates that earthy matter arising from heat has consumed the more subtle matter so that the earthy matter becomes partly *mixed with green,* because through the admixture of earthy and fiery matter a greenish color results. *If indeed the nails are not discolored,* or rather if no discoloration appears in the nails, this indicates that there is no inflammation in the organs of respiration capable of producing such a greenish color in the nails. But if even a slight tinge of green is present *other organs may be involved* in causing the staining of the nails, because such greenness may derive from the liver rather than from the trustworthy heart, the *seat of hope* and health which never fails. Even the greenness bursting forth from the liver does not originate in as great a fury of matter as does the lividity bursting forth from the heart; therefore this sign is merely symptomatic because true greenness arises from the heart's furor, whereas the other arises from the power of the liver to cleanse itself of superfluities (**56**).

17. *Additional signs should be noted:* the author told us above that a greenish discoloration of the nails is a mortal sign because it indicates inflammation arising in the part entrusted with life, but it should be noted that if before the green color is observed in the nails an easy action of respiration is noted, this indicates a healthy disposition of the heart, and then indeed the sign does not necessarily suggest death, and this is why he says *it is necessary to weigh all the signs,* favorable as well as unfavorable, in order to judge the expectancy of life or death. *For if the patient appears to be bearing up well* so that to a moderate degree he appears capable of sustaining his illness, *and other favorable symptoms develop,* such as an easy action of respiration, all this is considered by Antonius Musa (**57**) to be beneficial *and prognostic of a favorable termination,* that is, of a complete restoration to health. These two signs are best in any illness: first is the sick man's ability to sustain his illness and the other is easy respiration. *Whenever there is an abscess pointing outwards,* whether it arises from furious or from crude matter, *and the dangerous discoloration in the aforementioned places does not disappear,* that is, the abnormal coloration of the nails, this raises the danger that the furious matter may

dissolve the nails so that they eventually fall off completely (**58**).

18. *If the testes and adjacent parts and so forth:* the author now intends to prognosticate about the appearance of the testes and penis because from their arrangement during acute fevers signs may be elicited regarding the prospect of life or death. (**59**) The structure of these members is supplied with an abundance of nerves, veins, and arteries from the very earliest development of an animal of the male gender. As the penis develops, the matter from the veins, arteries, and nerves comes together and coalesces in the essence of one substance to constitute another definite subordinate member which lies adjacent to and below the penis (**60**), and it is from this member that the vital animal spirit is sent forth to inflame the penis and to cause it to become enlarged. If indeed the penis appears unduly small this may be caused by a loss of spirit, as in the spasm of inanition when such a loss occurs, or from an abscess arising in a principal part. For when an abscess arises in a principal part the testes and penis being exposed parts and on the body's surface relinquish spirit and heat to assist the noble part (**61**), and because those spirits which produce enlargement of the penis are lacking this organ appears unduly small, and this is what he teaches.

If the testes and penis appear unusually small, that is, if the diminution seems unnatural, *and they appear retracted,* this condition may result from a disturbance of the nerves so that those parts with which the nerves are connected become retracted. Such retraction also occurs from consumption of the substantial humidity and indicates spasm from inanition. *You may certainly expect pain and possibly death,* for in fact, diminution of these organs indicates the presence of an abscess, retraction indicates spasm from inanition which cannot be cured, and in fact, from excessive heat there is a consumption of the humors and a loss of those spirits with which the soul of the body is so closely enmeshed. When these spirits are lost completely, the soul is separated from the heart and death ensues.

19. [*Prognostics X*] *The patient's sleep should conform to habit:* every prognostic sign arises either from the body's form, from its actions or from its superfluities (**62**). The author previously pointed out signs to be inferred from the body's form; now he intends to discuss signs which may be inferred from the body's actions, and more precisely from the position assumed during sleep. Sleep is a period of rest for the animal powers and of renewed strength for the natural powers, in other words, during sleep the animal powers become inactive, though not entirely; but the power of vision is especially said to be at rest. The natural powers include appetite, digestion, nourishment, and elimination, and when food and drink pass through the triple stages of digestion, there

is a great release of fumes which seek the brain as if it were the furnace of the entire body. By stretching the membranes and moistening them the fumes compress the brain and narrow its channels to such an extent that the brain is weakened by successive dilatation and compression. With such constriction of the channels the spirit of vision cannot proceed to the eyes to stimulate the animal power of sight, and as a result sleep is induced, for at night heat is recalled to the interior of the body. This is not so by day, because the soul then detaches itself from the exterior parts in order to perform certain actions or operations, and expanding interiorly, thins out the humor and refines the gross spirits. Because these spirits are instruments of power, when they are refined they incite the virtues to a better performance of their duties. The natural heat itself when intensified also strengthens the virtues, and especially the animal virtues.

Sleep is correctly called the rest period of the animal virtues and so forth, and may be considered in regard to quantity, quality, and time of day. As regards quantity sleep may be excessive, diminished, or average: prolonged sleep arises from an excess of food and drink, by which many fumes are released, or it may arise from excessive humidity dominating the brain, as is seen in lethargy, or as a result of occlusion of the ventricles of the brain when the spirit becomes incapable of progressing along the continuity of the channels to the eyes.

False sleep is induced by and accompanies mortification, as may be observed in those taking opium (63). Loss of sleep may be attributed to a small intake of food and drink, to dryness of the brain as in phrenitis, or to pain, because pain produces an intensification of the catarrhal discharges with the result that the humors concentrate at the painful area, causing dryness and stinging.

Sleep should also be considered as to quality, because it may be sound or troubled. Sound sleep implies a favorable disposition of the brain and its coverings; troubled sleep a bad disposition of the brain and its coverings. Sleep should also be considered with respect to the time of day, because natural sleep occurs at night. Obscurity of vision has a collective or blurring effect, while clarity has a separative or dispersive effect (64). The cold of night leads heat back to the inner parts, and such heat, returned to the inner parts, releases fumes and induces sleep. The natural time of wakefulness is during the day, when clarity of vision has a separative effect and it is at this time that the soul detaches itself from the exterior parts to perform the activities of the waking hours which follow closely, but sleep which continues from early morning until nine should not be considered harmful, because these are the sanguine hours, and fumes are released from the overheated blood which induce sleep; the meaning is clear.

20. [*Prognostics XI*] *Evacuation of stool and so forth:* having set down the signs derived from the form of the body and from its actions as related to the nature of the digestive power, Hippocrates now intends to point out those signs which may be inferred from the superfluities which accompany the digestive process. First he prognosticates about the superfluities of the first digestion which is properly called elimination; and he prognosticates about this first with respect to the bad signs; then with respect to the more evil signs and finally with respect to the worst signs (65).

Elimination is considered in various ways: as to quantity, quality, time of day, number of evacuations, thinness or thickness of the stool, and mode of exit. As to quantity elimination may be large, small, or average, the first two occurring naturally or symptomatically. A large stool occurs naturally when nature, having well digested and subdivided matter, expels it through an evacuation, and by such an evacuation the patient is made to feel easier and more comfortable, indeed he is restored to health. A large stool may occur symptomatically, the quantity and quality being related to looseness of the parts, as may be seen in dysentery, a condition described in my glosses on the *Aphorisms* (66).

A small stool results when nature, having well digested and subdivided matter, expels it through other channels, leaving only a small residue in the intestines so that the evacuation is small, but by such an evacuation the patient is made to feel easier and more comfortable, indeed is restored to health. A small stool may develop symptomatically when excessive heat changes the feces into scyballa and this may bring on mania as Galen tells us in the case of a certain constipated man who was given a clyster which was retained with much pain. Finally Galen, by the use of emollient ointments, succeeded in causing a relaxation of the pudic circle so that the patient evacuated a sort of blackish substance. He states that when the same patient took food he returned it by vomit (67).

The quality of the stool is considered with respect to color, odor, thinness and thickness. If the stool is light yellow in color and semi-solid in consistency this is a laudable sign because it indicates the presence in moderation of both humors which are transmitted to the intestines and stomach, namely, phlegm and bile. Phlegm is transmitted to the stomach to aid the expulsive power and is sent thence to the intestines so that by its softening action it may aid the expulsive power in the release of feces. Bile is sent to the stomach to strengthen the appetite, and is then sent further on to the intestines so that by its gripping action it may assist in the abdomen's customary function. Phlegm does not predominate in the eliminated fecal matter to the extent that a whitish color becomes evident, nor does the bile predominate to the extent that a yellow color becomes evident, but from mutual interreaction, a composite color develops, namely, light yellow. Such a stool also indicates mildness of the active qualities of cold and heat, for obviously heat does not predominate sufficiently to produce the black color of burning nor does cold prevail sufficiently to produce whiteness, but from a mutual interreaction, a composite color develops. Such a stool also indicates the temper of the passive qualities, namely, dryness and humidity. Dryness does not predominate to such an extent that the stool becomes excessively hard in its movement towards the outlet, nor does humidity prevail so much that an excessive looseness results in a diarrhea, but from their mutual interreaction the stool remains semisolid. Again, if the stool is yellowish in color this indicates the presence of bile; if white, of phlegm; if red, of blood; if leaden-gray, of severe inflammation; if greenish, of gangrene; and if the color is black this indicates some combination of the preceding.

If the odor of the stool is fetid beyond ordinary this indicates corruption of the humors in a vital member. With respect to thinness and thickness, a thin liquid stool indicates abundance of the subtle humors, a thick stool, of the solid humors. The time of evacuation is considered because this should normally take place in mid-evening after digestion has been completed or at some other habitual hour. The frequency of elimination should be considered because if too frequent by reason of poor digestion the body's nourishment will be impaired. Finally, the act of elimination itself should be considered, for if the stool is passed with much noise this should be judged abnormal because it indicates weakness of heat and inability to eliminate the flatulence resulting from improper digestion.

In the evacuated stool any superfluity bears witness to a strong or weak disposition of the part in which it is generated. The stool, although it may then be called by another name, is first generated in the stomach and intestines, whence Hippocrates states that it attests to the strength or weakness of these organs. *In the evacuated stool* the substance eliminated is called "feces." *If the feces are not too dry* because of the absence of destructive dryness, *or [not] too liquid* and windy because of deficiency of the watery humors, but uniform in consistency, that is, in a semisolid state, *and if they are eliminated at the customary hour*, all this assures us that the body is not much altered from its earlier state. *This is a sign that the bowels are in a healthy state*, and the fact that the stool is not greasy is also a *good sign* because the fat of the body is not being lost by stool.

The author has prognosticated about satisfactory digestion, now he intends to talk about less favorable signs, such as a too liquid stool, because this indicates excessive heat producing a diarrhea accompanied by a watery elimination which cannot always be considered desirable, *and normal evacuation should occur without noise* or wind, because the natural heat has the power of absorbing the superfluous wind. *If the bowels do not move at a regular time this is a bad sign*, because a regular movement begins and ends without noise but an irregular movement begins first with noise and then continues without noise. *A too frequent movement is bad* because by such repeated eliminations or flux *the patient becomes weakened through overexertion*. It is extremely exhausting for a patient to be constantly going to stool because of an excessive flux, because from such a flux there results a complete loss of spirits and humors so that food prepared for the nourishment of the parts does not reach them *and loss of sleep results* because of this impairment of nutrition. By such a flux the body becomes impoverished from lack of food, dryness results, followed by sleeplessness, and this may lead the sufferer to a more serious condition because there is a complete loosening of the bonds by which the soul is enmeshed within the body.

It is desirable that the size of the stool be in proportion to the quantity of food consumed so that when much food is consumed, much is eliminated. But it should be noted that there are many foods which have a close affinity with the human system and are absorbed by the parts, so that a small elimination results; and on the other hand there are foods which are inimical to the system, and even when a small quantity of such foods is consumed there will be a large elimination. *Two or three times daily:* because perfect digestion cannot be repeated daily unless the waste material is evacuated two or three times. *But only once at night*, because with complete, repeated daily digestion there is little waste generated at night and one elimination suffices. *Just before dawn*, because this is the time when the sanguine humor predominates and a certain fume is released from the blood which assists the natural forces so that a satisfactory elimination results. *And according to his normal habit*, for this indicates the degree of exhaustion, and he should adhere to his normal habit because habit is second to nature.

As the disease comes to an end it is good for the diarrhea to clear up and the stool to become firm so that there may be a normal, regular bowel movement, of moderate size and consistency, indicating a blending of the passive qualities, namely dryness and humidity. The color should be yellowish, for this color indicates moderation of the bilious and phlegmatic humor, as well as moderation of the qualities of cold and heat; but lest anyone think that the stool ought to become solid and very firm, he advises against too much firmness because a very solid stool indicates strong, destructive heat.

21. *If round worms are eliminated with the stool* this is a favorable sign because it shows that the natural heat

which can transform the humors into animate life is strong (68), and this heat acting upon the humors near the surface covers them over as crust covers bread in the oven. The potential heat and the accidental heat which lie in the interior dissolve the humor into fumes, because when they are thoroughly dissolved the fumes acquire a greater subtility and can bring about the generation of a natural spirit. That spirit seeks an exit, but cannot leave because of the position of the surrounding crust and as a result a generation of worms occurs. Such a generation results from various kinds of phlegm, but not from bile whose bitterness kills the worms, nor from black bile which also has deadly qualities, nor from blood because, as our author states, when blood is unnaturally abundant in the abdomen it is changed into sanies. Generation, however, results either from salty phlegm and these worms are long and round because of long continuing heat, and round because of excessive dryness; or it may result from sweet phlegm, and these worms are long and broad, long from continuing heat and broad from humidity which causes them to spread laterally; and indeed these worms are worst, for those patients who have them in their wombs believe these worms to be serpents (69). If created from bitter phlegm worms are short and round because cold curtails their size and the dryness makes them round. Worms created from natural phlegm are short and broad: short from the cold which curtails their size and broad from humidity which produces spreading. Worms may assume various forms, depending upon the location in which they are distributed throughout the intestines: some are generated in the jejunum, others in the cecum, still others are scattered about in various parts of the intestine (70).

22. *In acute diseases the abdomen should not be too full:* that is, not too full of evil humors, but rather half empty, showing that the evil humors have been expelled. But because some may confuse emptiness after evacuation with loss of flesh, our author adds that the patient ought not to become *lean* or *wasted,* but *should retain flesh* in accordance with his usual appearance. *It is favorable to find a watery stool, but if the feces become too liquid* this indicates an impairment of digestion and the presence of a superabundance of subtle humors with the result that any medication administered to the patient is unable to adhere effectively. A liquid stool may develop from bile or black bile for even though some humors are dry and others are wet, all are substantially humid. Again he states that either *a white stool,* which indicates a cold humor conducive to the highest degree of impairment of digestion (for just as a white urine indicates a high degree of impairment of digestion, so does a stool of the same color), or *a very deep yellow* which indicates the beginning of inflammation, or *frothy stools* are all of evil significance. Every frothy

stool with the color of a hot humor suggests the onset of madness, whereas a similar stool with the color of a cold humor implies only an impairment of digestion or an admixture of flatulence.

It is also bad if the stool is small because this indicates a poor functioning of the lower parts due to inflammation, *or thick* because of added dryness, *or light in weight* because it contains fluid, *or white* which indicates impaired digestion, or *lemon-yellow* from intense heat, *or frothy* because the black color implies either inflammation or destruction; a green color developing from the preceding implies an inflammation, a leaden-blue color implies death of a part. *If the stool is fetid* this suggests corruption of a humor, *or green,* this announces the onset of inflammation, or *varicolored,* this indicates from the variety of colors a protracted illness with an excess of humors; *nor is this a less fatal sign,* for such a stool indicates inevitable destruction, *than the stool which carries off the scrapings of the intestines,* such as is seen in the first variety of dysentery, having the *color of leeks.* If the destruction results from severe inflammation then green bile is present in the case, *but a black stool is also dangerous* for the reason just mentioned (71). *It happens occasionally that all these colors appear simultaneously* because there may be superabundance of humors in a certain case, and this is a very bad sign because green alone announces danger, and this is here compounded by the presence of black, lemon-yellow and white.

23. *Flatulence and so forth:* our author has already discussed the gross superfluities of the first digestion, commonly known as the stool; now he intends to prognosticate about the fine superfluity of the first digestion, called flatulence. The superfluity of the first digestion may be either gross or fine, depending on the strength or weakness of heat, weak heat acting on fine superfluity being sufficient to dissolve and absorb it but not to eliminate it. The dissolved superfluity seeks an exit but meets with resistance from the outside air so that after dashing from one side to another it finally makes an exit through the narrow passage and produces a sound. Likewise a strong heat acting on a gross superfluity dissolves it into an excess of fine superfluities which then seek an exit but meet with resistance from the air and finally make their exit with a sound. Moderate heat working on gross superfluities dissolves as much as is required to break down the digested matter and modify it to a normal thickness. It then naturally exists without sound. Therefore it is better to pass stool without sound through the action of moderate heat than with sound, because this indicates excessive strength or weakness of heat, as has been said.

To pass flatulence without sound is best: you must understand, however, that while it is better than with sound *nevertheless it is better that elimination should occur with sound than that flatulence be retained,* for if the retained fumes seek an exit and cannot be removed through the inferior parts they are rushed to the superior parts where they mingle with the organs of breathing and, being unable to free themselves, are sent to the brain. Thus the brain is irritated and weakened in its actions, and *this is a warning sign of delirium*, for indeed madness results from stretching a certain part of the brain and pain results from such an impairment of continuity. *He is in severe pain unless he voluntarily retains the flatulence:* this may happen when one is in fine company and cannot expel the gas so that it is voluntarily retained and returns to the hypochondria to cause pain. Therefore in referring to these matters he says: *pain in the hypochondria has this character* or nature: if the pain is of recent origin, arising unexpectedly from flatulence *and without a rise in heat*, then one can be certain that the pain does not originate from warm matter which is readily carried off, but the word "recent" applies to newly created cold matter which produces pain of long duration. *If a rumbling noise occurs*, this heralds the movement of flatulence and feces to the exit and *elimination* by stool. But when the matter to be eliminated is excessive it may be excreted at times by stool, at other times by urine, for the abdomen possesses these two methods of elimination. However, at times there is so much flatulence in the abdomen that it cannot be eliminated completely by stool or urine but descends to the scrotum (**72**), causing this organ to swell, but being sieve-like the flatulence disappears; or it may descend further through the third branch of the chylous vein to the feet causing them to swell and to become dropsical, and then the flatulence disappears; *in general, flatulence is transmitted to lower parts of the body.*

24. [Prognostics XII] *That urine is best and so forth:* the author has already prognosticated about both superfluities of the first digestion, namely the gross and the fine (**73**). Now he proposes to prognosticate about the superfluity of the second digestion, or urine, discussing dropsy as well. He therefore praises healthy urine which by presenting a good sediment demonstrates the demarcation between what is dissolved and undissolved. For as Isaac says, each part has a prefixed and determined end so that it performs a definite function which no other part is capable of performing. From this we understand that no single part can make up for the imperfection of another, so that if the third digestion is good, the preceding second and first were also good, and if the first digestion is bad, then the second and third will be bad. In this connection it should be noted that all-powerful and provident nature has prepared certain parts by which food may be grasped and skillfully prepared for transformation, these being the mouth and stomach.

Food is chewed up in the mouth but is not sufficiently altered for digestion in this manner. It was

ordained that the stomach be of a white color and that for its activity there be provided a subtle substance of a cold and dry nature. Food arriving at the stomach is changed, regardless of previous color, to white by this subtle substance and is prepared to move on, but such motion is delayed by cold and dry qualities which have a centripetal motion. If we consider other organs we shall find none of an identical nature, so that if poor digestion occurs in the stomach this fault cannot be made good by another organ.

The liver is a warm, humid organ, purple in color (purple being composed of red, black, and a trace of white) and has an earthy substance. No other organ of the body has exactly this composition, so that if digestion is performed poorly in the liver it will be poor in all other organs as well (**74**). Indeed the process of digestion finally terminates in the four basic discharges of the body, for when digestion is a natural act it terminates in the basic discharges, and any natural act is completed in three stages, namely, beginning, middle, and final.

If the final stage is good then the entire process was good, so that if the third digestion is good so is its superfluity, and if the superfluity is good so is the blood, and if the blood is good so is its substance. And if this substance is good then so was the action by which it was generated, and because it was generated through the second digestion then this was also good and its superfluity is good, so that when the urine is good so is its sediment.

In the sediment three things are principally to be looked for, although a fourth is said to be allied to these. Principally one should pay attention to clarity of color, the disposition of the sediment at the fundus and the continuity of the substance in assuming the form of a pine cone. The fourth, which is allied to these, is regularity in passing urine, that is to say, in urinating at regular intervals. During the period under observation a sediment of white color is laudible, and indicates the performing of an orderly routine activity and the completion of the process of the third digestion. For it was necessary that the sediment be changed from its original form and freed from the blood which tinged it red at the beginning of the transformation. Then through the interchange of parts as well as from the boiling heat the original appearance is changed, the urine assumes an aqueous appearance and there is no trace of blood in the superfluity, or hypostasis, for water being an element which seeks in every way possible to pass into the earth, it was necessary to change the blood into a white color before it was prepared to pass into parts whose essence is earthy. This continuity of substance indicates the successful completion of local activity occurring during the third digestion.

Such a transposition was needed because these parts were improperly arranged, nor indeed did this interchange indicate any fault in the virtue of the blood because it was destroyed by the heat. Fumes pushing forward or separating violently from the force of the heat assume a pineate form because natural heat begins with a motion from the center, and after swirling rapidly around some object begins to spread laterally before elongating and projecting to a point, much in the manner of a flame, and heat naturally corresponds to a flame because it also begins with a lateral spreading, and so on (75). In this way, according to the Greeks, fire (which they call "pir") arises as may be seen in a piece of coal pointed at the top and spreading laterally below, and from this word is derived "piramides," the burial places of the ancients. Terrestrial heat combined with its own watery sediment settles down and finds a position at the lower part. Airy, subtle substances lie above while the fiery particles assume the highest position in the fundus, thus indicating successful completion of the required motion. It was necessary that both form and substance be altered in order to effect such a passage. The terrestrial parts change blood into earthiness so that not only blood itself but its superfluity acquires this earthiness and therefore seeks the fundus.

Regularity of time of urination is considered: this should be maintained with few variations until the disease is ready to terminate on a critical day. The continuance of such variations indicates a perfect action of the third digestion and the continued effectiveness of the second digestion.

That urine is good which has a white sediment: such urine is rightly considered good because it has the proper color and substance, and being in a perfect state indicates that the third digestion has been successfully performed in the various parts, and if the third digestion is good, then so were the first and second. It has the proper color, that is, only slightly reddish, thus indicating an evenness of the passive qualities. Why then is a white color praised in the urinary sediment although considered objectionable elsewhere in nature? Because having been freed of its color the earthy portion of the urine settles down and becomes stationed at the fundus, and because earthy particles, being naturally somewhat weighty, also seek the fundus. *And remains uniform,* that is, this uniformity of color persists and does not vary from one day to another. Or as others say, *it should be uniform one day after another and continuous* because of absence of flatulence, *and light,* or free of particles, *and unvarying,* when there is a simple continuation of the color, or variable when urine which was dark at the beginning of a disease does not retain this color until the crisis. *And if it remains thus until the crisis,* that is, if there is persistence of the good qualities in the urine *until the crisis,* that is, until the decline of the disease, such a termination is favorable because it derives from natural vigor. *This is a definite sign of improvement* resulting from natural

vigor and satisfactory digestion. Vigor of the natural powers and satisfactory digestion indicate strength of natural heat, and natural heat revives the virtues. For the nature of similar things is changed equally by the nature of their functions so that there is hope of recovery.

But if the urine continues at times with a sediment as just described and at other times without such sediment, it indicates an illness of long duration for it indicates a weakness of nature which at times is capable of expelling the superfluities, but not at other times. When nature is weakened, or even before, the patient begins to fail as the strength of the disease prevails and indeed when sufficiently debilitated, he succumbs, but this sign is not entirely reliable, and may place the physician in doubt.

25. *A urine which is excessively red in color:* the author indicated above that a good urine with a good sediment signifies shortness of the disease. Now he intends to show that a less favorable urine, with a sediment similar to itself, indicates a protracted illness. A deep redness persisting in the urine and sediment indicates that an excess of blood is tinging the substance and sediment of the urine. Because of this excess of blood the illness will linger on because such an excess of matter cannot be digested in a short time; nevertheless, because blood is a digestible humor and friendly to human nature it signifies that the illness will end well. *Urine which is excessively red,* that is, deep red, *with a sediment of a similar color,* that is, deep red or somewhat lighter, *indicates a more protracted illness than the previous one* because a large quantity of blood is harmful and prolongs the illness. *Nevertheless this is still a sure and safe sign of eventual recovery,* for it denies the presence of a raging febrile humor, or an unpurified one, but attests to the presence of a sanguine humor which is warm and humid and has life-giving qualities. It aids digestion by these qualities and is readily dispersed through various parts of the body.

If the sediment is coarse: a coarse sediment which varies from white to red indicates liquefaction of the parts and eventual dissolution; a blood-red color indicates severe destruction. Such charred blood being less suitable for digestion indicates a more protracted illness. A coarse sediment with urine which is persistently red has a bad prognosis because it indicates the second variety of hectic fever which is incurable (76). By this time the heat is so implanted in the various parts that it consumes the body's humidity throughout its length and breadth. The worst variety is flaky urine because this indicates a major dissolution. Flaky particles in the urine arise from the bladder because the bladder, being white and concave, the scales are similarly concave and white, and if the heat is too strong it has the power to dissolve the bladder into scales, although this organ is cold, hard, and accessible. This occurs internally where heat properly increases in strength as well as in those members which are naturally warm and soft and have lost all their humidity. Moreover, the sediment may be white and liquid, a superfluity of the third digestion. Here by the term "sediment" we refer to the phlegmatic humors which appear in the lower part of the urine because anything which is heavy by nature seeks the lower parts. If phlegmatic humors appear in the urine they indicate the presence of cold matter which requires a long time for digestion. *Therefore if the sediment is white* because of the persistence of phlegmatic humors, *and liquid*, that is, clear, *this is a bad sign* because the matter must be unusually difficult to digest, but even worse than this is a sediment full of scales, because it indicates that the firmer parts are being dissolved.

26. *White clouds suspended in the urine and so forth:* it must be noted that the sediment of the third digestion has three designations depending on its location. At the bottom, it is called "ypostasis," from "ypos" meaning "below" and "stasis," "remaining"; in the center, it is called "emorroyda," which means "hanging down"; and at the surface, it is called "nephilis" or "cloud," from its resemblance to clouds. It should be noted also that any one of these sediments may be termed a cloud, or a cloudy body, because it obscures the substance of the urine. A white sediment at the base is best; when suspended in the center this is not so good; and a white cloud at the surface is by far the most harmful. A black sediment at the base is a most evil sign; it is less evil when suspended in the center; and still less evil when it appears at the surface.

A white sediment is best because it indicates completion of the third digestion by which the blood is decolorized as it rightly should be. If the superfluity of the blood is of the same color as the blood itself, this is a very good sign; but when a white sediment is in suspension this is not so good, because it indicates that the substance in suspension has not settled downward. If elevated at the surface this is bad because it indicates the presence of wind generated as a result of weakness of the natural heat, because the heat has not had sufficient strength to destroy the wind. A white cloud indicates much less danger, even though there is a larger accumulation of wind, because it signifies the heart's ability to raise the sediment to the surface; for the greater the accumulation of wind, the greater the weakness of the natural heat.

A black sediment is a most evil sign because it indicates burning or mortification of the earthy matter; when preceded by a green color it indicates burning; by a leaden color, mortification. A black suspension is less harmful because there is less earthy matter in the suspension than in the sediment, thus indicating a lesser degree of burning and mortification A black cloud at the surface by virtue of the refinement of the matter indicates only the onset of burning and mortification, and is therefore far less to be feared.

A cloud suspended in the urine: here "nebula" is interpreted in a broad sense as "ypostasis," because the entire body of the urine is cloudy, and *suspended* means "clearly visible." *If white it is good* because it indicates the greatest good, *if black it is bad* because it indicates the greatest danger; *while a yellow and clear urine indicates impairment of digestion during the course of the illness* and the presence of undigested matter. It must be noted that urine may become tinged not only by extraneous heat but also by natural heat. As Constantinus says, extraneous heat alone may produce a discoloration in the urine by preparing matter unsuitable for digestion through absorption and rarefaction; but on the other hand if the natural heat is weak and finds the matter already prepared, it continues in its own way and adds to the fiery particles consumed. For we see that anyone by cutting up tough meats with a knife makes them suitable for cooking, so that even weak heat becomes adequate.

A light yellow urine persisting in any illness indicates weakness of natural heat which cannot improve itself, for if unable to effect a change at the beginning and in the early stages of the disease when there is still strength of some sort, it will be far less able to effect a change when the patient is weaker, so that when such a fever continues over a very long period of time the patient succumbs. And such urine, if produced through dryness, causes this dryness to be carried throughout all the solid parts so that the humors become thickened and impairment of digestion persists, *so that we must fear for the patient's life* in those cases where nature is weakened by a protracted illness. *Aqueous urine is indicative of death:* by watery urine is meant colorless urine, because "aquosa" is so called from "aqua" or "water," and such colorless urine arising at the onset of an illness is a faithful and certain herald of death, because it signifies a long, protracted illness with eventual loss of the patient. However, if urine is scanty and unfavorable signs persist the outlook is also bad, as we can see in phrenesis, because this means that there is retention of the harmful matter while the natural heat is being extinguished. If there is a good flow of urine at the end of an illness with persistence of favorable signs the outlook is good, because this indicates that the harmful matter has been dissolved and eliminated.

Fetid urine is bad because it indicates that the natural heat is weak and incapable of purging the patient of his impurities, and because what the warm humor dissolves the natural heat should destroy. When impurities accumulate and are not eliminated they give off an odor which alters the urine so that it becomes fetid. A fetid odor indicates corruption of the humors and a tendency toward putridity, and this may be considered *a faithful sign* of death.

Black urine is bad because it indicates burning or mortification, and *fatty urine is bad* because it indicates an excess of the solid humors crowding into the urine. This sign is equally dangerous in both sexes so that he emphasizes that it is very serious, not only in men but in both men and women. Among the colors mentioned green is by far the worst in men because it indicates severe inflammation; black preceded by a leaden color is worst in women because it indicates mortification. *In children, a watery urine is particularly bad*, some say because it indicates a complete alteration in the two qualities especially concerned with care of this age group, namely heat and humidity (**77**).

A watery or oily *quality* of the urine is also bad in children because it indicates that the matter is unstable and that the child is about to waste away. *A urine* which is *clear* or thin and a urine which is *thick* or white and *prolonged* over an unusual period time, even though accompanied by other signs of free and easy inspiration and expiration, may be a *certain indication of the future development of a subdiaphragmatic abscess*, that is, an abscess in those parts concerned with nutrition. For a white color arises from increasing cold in the aqueous parts and aqueous humors, so that a white urine indicates an excess of cold humors causing it to be thin, and this indicates that dryness is working toward a thickening of the humors with the result that the illness is protracted and the patient becomes weakened. With such weak forces he is unable to go through a crisis, and because the pendent matter is heavy from the cold and thickens of itself it has a tendency to settle at a lower point rather than a higher, and thus is more apt to collect under the diaphragm than above.

Oily deposits which resemble spider webs floating on the urine are an ominous sign (**78**), for they indicate a dissolution of the fatty matter so that according to our author, *this sign indicates that the patient is about to waste away* or be dissolved. *One must not neglect to observe the position and arrangement of the "cloud,"* for there are three positions to be noticed in the sediment: the lower, middle, and upper. The first mentioned sediment may be called "nebula" or "cloud," because by its interposition it makes the urine cloudy, so that we may speak of "nebula" in place of "ypostasis," although the latter is the correct term; *and whether the cloud is placed at the bottom or top*, that is, whether it is in the middle of the urine-glass or below; *and the uniformity of color*, because a white cloud in the middle and a colored one elsewhere is a bad sign, while such a development in the upper zone is of even worse significance. *Whereas a white cloud in the middle, with the upper zone of the aforementioned color*, that is white, *is very good*, or at least much less dangerous than a white cloud in the center *with black at the upper zone, for this is extremely dangerous*, although black in the lower zone

is also dangerous because of inflammation of the earthy parts.

One must observe whether the bladder itself is not affected, for at times, a scaly sediment arises from the bladder itself, at other times from an involvement of the body as a whole. Our author teaches us how to distinguish these conditions (**79**). Flakiness coming from the bladder itself has a thick substance, whereas flakiness originating in the body as a whole has a thin substance. *The physician should therefore take heed* lest he be misled into diagnosing a disordered condition of the bladder because such a defect in the bladder is very serious, when similar defects may originate, as he says, in other parts of the body, *or when the defect does occur in this particular organ, to think that it originates elsewhere*, for in the latter case the sediment is lighter and indeed this is his precise explanation.

27. [*Prognostics XIII*] *That vomitus is most useful:* the author now intends to prognosticate about vomited matter, that is, about anything which is brought up through vomiting (**80**). The subject is considered in various ways: as to quantity, quality, and time; as to quantity because there may be much or little, and both quantities may occur naturally or symptomatically. A profuse vomitus occurs naturally when some harmful matter attacks the upper region of the organs of nutrition, and is expelled from the entire body by vomiting, and by such an expulsion the sick man is made to feel easier and more comfortable. A small quantity is natural when nature almost completely expels the offending substance through the lower regions so that little remains in the superior parts, hence there is a small vomitus. A profuse vomitus may occur symptomatically either from the quality of the matter or its fury, or it may arise from an excessive quantity of matter so that the vomiting is abundant and thick, or from lack of control within the organs so that they become engorged with matter, with the result that foodstuffs when ingested are rejected. A small vomitus may occur symptomatically when the matter is so violent and rarified that when ejected it seeks the upper parts with the result that there is a small vomitus.

As to quality, it may be considered with regard to color, odor, taste, thinness and thickness. The first color to be considered is light yellow: this is praised because it indicates an evenness of the two active qualities, namely heat and cold, which in turn control the two humors naturally proceeding to the stomach, namely phlegm and bile. Again yellow indicates an excess of bile and so forth. Odor is considered because a fetid odor indicates a corruption of the humors, while a heavy odor implies the beginning of corruption of the humors. Smell is also considered because if the vomitus has a vinegary smell this indicates the presence of black bile or sour phlegm and so forth. Both thinness and thickness are considered because if the vomitus is refined and thin this indicates an abundance of the refined and fluid humors; if thick, of the gross humors. As to time one should observe whether the vomitus occurs on a critical day. The author states: *that vomitus is most useful in which phlegm is mixed with bile,* that is, one which arises from an admixture of phlegm and bile in such proportions that bile does not predominate sufficiently to produce a saffron color, or phlegm a white color, but from their mutual interreaction a yellow color appears.

And is not too viscid, but rather of a medium consistency, indicating an even temper of the passive qualities with the result that rarifying dryness does not predominate to such an extent as to produce a very thin matter or humidity so as to produce a very thick matter. *Now just as most cases are quite removed from this ideal state of simplicity,* that is, from a simple nature possessing no harmful qualities (in the same way as we speak of a simple man), *and are distant indeed from this ideal simplicity,* or from such an unusual and peculiar state of innocence, so much more must we be on guard when the cases show no evidence of temperance or of moderation. *For there may be vomitus resembling the juice of leeks,* thus indicating the onset of inflammation, *or greenish,* still greater destruction, *or lead-colored,* the onset of mortification, *or blackish,* indicating either mortification or severe inflammation. *If the vomitus is tinged with all these colors this is a fatal sign,* indicating that contrary humors have a hold on the stomach, such as reddish bile; or a variety of colors may result from the contrary action of overabundant qualities. When all these colors mentioned above appear together they herald destruction, indeed, they announce the individual's death. *Any pain which persists is bad,* and if accompanied by a vomitus which has a heavy or fetid odor indicates a harmful development of dire significance.

28. [*Prognostics XIIII*] *Sputum in all acute diseases and so forth:* the author now intends to prognosticate about the sputum. Sputum is assigned to certain parts to be excreted, namely, the brain, stomach, and lung. When leaving the brain it departs with a blowing noise; from the lung it is discharged by expectoration or coughing; and from the stomach it is excreted naturally so that sputum may be emitted from any one of these three organs. It is most properly emitted from the lung, where there is in fact an excessive generation of phlegm, because the lung itself is cold and humid. During the second digestion the lung draws this cold to itself for the generation of phlegm, Sputum therefore is an indication of disease in the lungs or its contingent parts, such as pleurisy or pneumonia (81). Pleurisy is an abscess arising in the delicate parts protected by the ribs; pneumonia is an abscess formed in close proximity to the lung, namely in the chasuble which

covers the lung, and is called "peripleumonia" from "pery," meaning "around," and "plegmio," meaning "lung," because the condition develops near the lung and not within its very substance as some seem to believe.

Sputum is considered in various ways: as to quantity, quality, time and manner of exit. It is considered as to quantity because in one case there may be much sputum, in another little, and such variations may occur naturally or symptomatically. Much sputum is produced naturally when harmful matter has been well digested and led forth from the body, and through such a discharge the patient is made to feel easier and more comfortable, or may even be restored to health. A small quantity is produced naturally when the harmful matter enters almost entirely into venous channels which carry it to the liver; it leaves the liver by the chylous duct which carries it to the kidneys where it is excreted with the urine. Much sputum is produced symptomatically either from the quantity of matter or from lack of control of the parts. Little sputum is produced symptomatically when there is mortification and inflammation or weakness of the expulsive virtue.

The quality of sputum is considered from several points of view, including color, odor, smell, thinness and thickness. As to color, there should at first be some pink mixed in with the healthy sputum, and by the seventh day, the appearance should change. A pinkish sputum is a favorable sign because it indicates that sanguine matter is passive to both qualities and is being changed into purulent matter for excretion. When blended with healthy sputum this indicates that the body has not been altered greatly from its earlier condition. The fact that from the seventh day onward the appearance of the sputum changes indicates that strength of the natural heat at the point of coction of the harmful matter is allied with strength of the digestive virtue. Again if a bright red color persists it indicates an abundance of blood, and so forth.

As to odor, a fetid odor is considered dangerous because it indicates corruption of the humors and a serious corruption of the parts. Odor is considered in sputum as it was in sweat. Sputum is also considered as to time because excretion ought to happen on a critical day, and as to the manner of exit, because it may proceed with difficulty, or without, as our author states.

Sputum in all diseases of the lung, as in pneumonia, *or of the chest,* as in pleurisy, *should be expectorated rapidly* because of the power of the expulsive virtue and easily because the matter lends itself readily to digestion, *and without exertion,* so that the crudity and viscosity are easily removed. And the inflammation should not be concentrated in one area so as to render the work of nature difficult, nor should the sputum be too thick. *If the sputum is pinkish in color,* this signifies digestion of the sanguine matter and blending with healthy sputum, indicating that the body has not been altered greatly from its earlier condition, but if the *expectoration is sluggish*, then the force of nature has been slowed down by viscosity, crudity, inflammation, or an excess of accumulated matter. *If pain occurs at the onset*, that is, in confirmation of the presence of an abscess, and increases in intensity, *this is a very bad sign*, because it indicates the violence of the matter, and such sputum remains *bright red* because the veins are stripped open by raging matter.

Or the sputum may be *light yellow*, indicating that the bile is overly heated, and accompanied by a *labored* cough, as when the patient is seen to cough and expel nothing; *and is not mixed with healthy sputum*, thus indicating that the body has indeed been altered considerably from its earlier condition. *A red sputum is extremely harmful* because it indicates rupture of veins in the lung; *white* indicates impaired digestion; *thick*, deep-seated dryness; *globular*, cold producing mortification; *green and frothy*, indicates inflammation; and *black, which is worst of all*, indicates mortification. *And if a rattling sound persists in the chest* because of cold causing mortification or because of deep-seated dryness, and *there is little or no expectoration, this is a fatal sign*, because it indicates the strength of deep-seated dryness which produces an ominous sound at the end of life, called the "death rattle."

29. *Sneezing with catarrh:* the author now prognosticates about sneezing. Sneezing is the sound produced by a violent commotion in the brain—such a violent commotion being associated with strength of the expulsive virtues and weakness of the retentive virtue, both persisting until the brain is moved to expel those superfluities with which it has been oppressed. *Sneezing with catarrh*, that is, with a catarrhal flow of the humors: catarrh means a flow of humor to some part of the body, and the flow of the catarrhal humor becoming fixed near the organs of breathing, the matter is collected into a pulmonic abscess. All pain aggravates this catarrhal flow and the humors run together to the painful area. *Sneezing with catarrh* occurs when there is a violent confluence of such catarrh-producing humors. *In all diseases of the lungs and chest*, as in pleurisy and pneumonia, *it is a bad sign* if matter fills the abscess so that through such continuous flow of the humors there is increased pain and accumulation of fluid with the result that there is ever more repletion with choking. *Whether sneezing begins before* the violent flow *or begins at the same time*, that is, accompanies the flow, *this is a bad sign* because it indicates violence of the catarrhal humor, flowing and being collected, and finally leading to the formation of an abscess. *But sneezing in other diseases without an accompanying catarrh*, or violent flux, is beneficial, for the brain being strong can expel those humors which collect to form an abscess so that sneezing results.

Our author has already said something about blood-tinged sputum, now he adds a few words on this subject. *Sputum which is pinkish and clear* and does not result from a disturbance of the humors indicates that it is mixed with healthy sputum, and this in turn indicates the sick man's ability to withstand his illness. *And if such sputum occurs at the onset of the lung disease it is a good sign*, because it indicates that the matter is amenable to both qualities of digestion. *But if such sputum lasts until the seventh day or longer* and remains unchanged *this is a suspicious sign*, because if at the beginning of the illness and with both qualities amenable to digestion, the patient could not completely digest the matter, now that he is weakened digestion will certainly be less effective.

All expectoration which does not result in the relief of pain is serious because it indicates the presence of matter which is so furious and plentiful that it spreads extensively by its violence and chokes off the breathing apparatus. *All pain in the aforementioned locations*, that is, in the lungs and costal regions, may be *followed by expectoration or looseness of the bowels: such looseness occurs* in the bowels when matter is being collected to form an abscess at the diaphragm, and as noted by Isaac in the *Viaticum* (82) this results in a false pleurisy. This matter is carried by the vessels to the stomach, is received into the concavity of the stomach and induces a looseness of the bowels. *If after phlebotomy or the administration of any indicated medicine* diuresis occurs *but the pain is not relieved* this gives warning of pus formation, because the matter is closed off and converted into pus.

Suppuration of a bilious nature: the author has already told us that all pain in the aforementioned regions accompanied by expectoration or looseness of the bowels but not followed by a decrease in pain must indicate the presence of pus. Now lest anyone think that every decrease in pus is good the author counters this idea by the present discussion of *suppuration of a bilious nature*, that is, one which is green or black in color and mixed with normal sputum. You must understand that when sputum appears by itself and is not accompanied by putrid bile it is an indication of health, but *it is bad* when the suppuration is green or black thus indicating a furious destructive quality, for by this desiccating fury the pus demolishes and destroys the parts. *And especially if the seventh day has already been reached:* for as he said earlier the appearance of putrid bile before the seventh day is not so much to be feared because natural heat, being vigorous at the onset of the disease, acts on the matter over a period of time and converts it into sanies, but if the natural heat was not strong enough at the onset or during the seven days to change the matter into sanies then this change will definitely not occur when he is in a much weaker condition.

If the natural heat which regulates the human body is weakened then the virtues are also weakened, so that the mechanism of the human body becomes a heavy load for the patient to support (83).

And you may fear death by the fourteenth day because of the increased severity of the illness, for if this putrid bile persists until the eleventh day by that time the matter has been present for so long a period as to weaken the patient, and you may anticipate death by the fourteenth day because the matter still remains very destructive and the patient is, by then, extremely weak. Now you must not simply predict death, *but in fact unless a favorable change occurs you must consider this condition fatal*, that is, unless a few favorable signs make their appearance in the usual manner; *one such favorable sign being strength* and self-possession of the patient, indicating some vitality of the natural heat. As a result crudity is lacking, having been removed from the matter, for the natural heat's strength is opposed to crudity of matter and this indicates a tempered abundance of the humors such as are opposed to the matter's violence. *Easy breathing*, that is, easy inspiration and expiration, occurs when the inflamed matter which causes choking is absent, for when there is no interference with the action of inspiration and expiration there is not much matter present to produce choking, but when choking does occur the breath fails. *And easy ejection of the putrid matter with cough:* because the expulsive virtue is so strong that the patient need not labor in expectorating and is not hindered by any contrary humor or humors, or by any contrary quality or qualities. *And there is equal warmth over the entire body as is natural*, that is, there is a favorable distribution of heat to the interior parts and to the surface, to the exposed and non-exposed members, to those which are noble and ignoble. By such an even distribution of heat fear of an abscess developing in the interior of the body is removed, because when the interior parts are in pain the warm spirit is drawn to the interior parts and the external parts become cold.

Warmth may vary from moderate to intense: the more intense heat dissolves and consumes to such a degree that an induration develops, whereas moderate heat by dissolving and consuming just as much as is needed causes a softness to predominate with resultant disappearance of the accidental heat. *Nor is there excessive thirst:* because there is no interference with nourishment; this indicates a good disposition of the liver and excellent functioning of the nutritive parts. *But there are bowel movements* which indicate good function and disposition of the stomach and intestines; *perspiration*, which indicates a favorable disposition of the entire body; and *sleep*, which indicates a favorable disposition of the animate parts. *All these signs are considered good*, that is, no matter how much these functions may be interfered with *they still give promise of life* and from them signs of future recovery

may be elicited. *If only a few of these signs are present this is bad*, that is, if there is a disappearance of several signs and the good signs remain fewer in number than they should be. Now when the favorable signs are lacking and the harmful ones predominate *you may be certain of a fatal termination* and that death will supervene because of the weakness of nature.

It should be noted whether there are as many good signs as bad, for if the good signs are more effectual then the bad health will return, but if the bad are more effectual the result will be death. *Adverse signs may predict death*, that is, there are adverse signs other than those mentioned above by which death may be predicted. *To be observed among these are the patient's weakness, deep and labored respiration, and thick profuse expectoration accompanied by a painful, persistent cough:* also because of weakness of the expulsive virtue thirst arises, but this may arise spontaneously as when there is a boiling over of bilious matter and the organs of breathing become so disturbed by the heat that the warm fumes dry the mouth of the stomach, thus producing thirst; or thirst may be present because of lack of nourishment. *Unequal warmth of the body* may result from the presence of an abscess developing in the interior parts when the external parts become cold in sympathy with the interior parts and the abdomen feels cold, *yet there is an excessive heat of the flanks* because of warm, heat-producing fumes. The forehead, hands, and feet are cold because heat is extinguished first in these parts, or to put it differently, heat relinquishes first those parts which it sought out last. Then *the urine* indicates a bad disposition of the stomach, and *the perspiration* indicates an imperfect digestion and a poor disposition of the entire body, and *the spleen* indicates a bad disposition of the animate members. All of these signs, as we have said, are menacing and predict *impending death*, that is, death in the very near future.

If the signs described above occur with the ejection of bilious matter this of itself is enough for destruction, *and death before the fourteenth day is not to be doubted, if it has not already occurred by the ninth*, by which time nature has already been greatly weakened, *or by the eleventh day* when nature has been more seriously weakened. *With such reflections you may determine mortality from the sputum*, that is after reflecting on the signs mentioned above; but if *there are signs of vitality*, that is, if by the use of logic you discover signs favoring life, *or you recognize prognostic signs of death you will proceed surely and accurately* and will then ascribe life to those who will survive and death to those who are about to die.

30. *Abscesses and so forth:* the author has already considered how various abscesses terminate within various periods but he did not introduce the exact time for their rupture or termination. Therefore

he now intends to indicate the exact time of rupture or termination of the abscesses, and intends to point out differences between the bilious, sanguine, phlegmatic, and atrabilious abscesses. The sanguine abscess postpones its rupture until some time before the twentieth day, because it has two qualities which act concordantly to break down matter, namely humidity and heat; the phlegmatic abscess postpones its rupture until the twentieth day, for although it possesses cold which is not in accord with dissolution of matter, it does possess humidity which is very powerful and is consistent with dissolution. The bilious abscess postpones its rupture until the fortieth day, for although it may possess one factor agreeable to dissolution, namely heat, nevertheless it also possesses dryness which is not at all consistent with dissolution. The atrabilious abscess postpones its rupture until the sixtieth day because both of its qualities are antagonistic to dissolution so that this does not occur quickly, and this is what he says.

Some abscesses break by the twentieth day, such as the sanguine abscess before the twentieth day and the phlegmatic abscess on the twentieth; *others break on the fortieth*, as the bilious abscess; *others continue to the sixtieth*, as the atrabilious abscess. *The physician must know the exact day of the beginning of suppuration* for as the assistant of nature the physician should not be uninformed, but must record the exact day of suppuration for various reasons, namely, to study the progress of the disease and to determine from the day of rupture whether the patient is suffering from a tertian or quartan fever. Having observed the signs of the dissolution of matter he can then deliver his medication on a critical day. But nature cannot always be watched in her diverse ways. Our author states this because there are various kinds of abscesses and their terminations occur at irregular times, and because of these variations the physician may be deceived.

It behooves the physician therefore to inform himself as to the exact day of onset of the abscess: one onset may precede the fever, another may begin with the fever, and still another may occur at the onset of the illness itself. If the onset of suppuration precedes the fever then in some unusual manner the sole antecedent cause already existed in the body at the very beginning of the illness. If suppuration begins with the onset of fever the disease becomes active when the body becomes warm or first experiences an unnatural chill. When the onset of suppuration occurs at the time of the fully developed illness this is postponed until the fourth day, persists until the eleventh, or at times until the sixteenth, and, according to Galen even to the hundredth day, and this is what he teaches. *It behooves the physician therefore to inform himself as to the exact day of onset of the abscess:* that is, the day of onset of the abscess, not the time of the fully developed illness, not the time of onset before

fever, but the exact date of onset with fever (**84**), and *in what hour the body first suffered unnaturally from chills and fever and when the patient first felt a piercing pain in that place.* From the racing around of the humor it is eventually collected to form an abscess.

Furthermore the physician must be familiar with the quality of the pain, whether it be localized, stabbing, very severe or widespread. If it is localized you may predict a termination on the twentieth day; if stabbing, on the fortieth; if very severe on the sixtieth. *These are the first signs of a collection of pus:* namely, chills and fever, but when matter is collected to form an abscess, pain also begins as the continuity is dissolved. All pain intensifies the catarrhal flow, the breath is disordered by overheating and thus the body becomes unnaturally warm. *And it is from that time,* that is, from the onset of the abscess, *that you must count in order to predict when the abscess will break,* whether on the twentieth or fortieth or sixtieth day.

Also consider whether the abscess is forming on only one side of the body, or, as may happen, on both. One must observe whether the abscess forms on one side of the body or both, *for if only one side is involved you will find it useful to examine further,* and you should search carefully as follows. *If on one side,* that is, of the upper *abdomen, there is noted a greater concentration of heat,* then we shall consider that the abscess is developing at that point, and that there is no abscess on the other side. *Order the patient to lie on one side* in order to see whether the site of the abscess is relieved, and *if there is an abscess on the other side* from the one on which he is lying *he will have a sensation of weight* from the racing of the humor to the site of that abscess. Now if he does not feel this heaviness *you may determine the side on which the abscess is located and also that both sides are not involved.* And there are still other signs of an abscess *by which you may determine which abscesses are of a putrid nature,* or, as he says, other evidence of abscess formation may be inferred from the following signs: *the fever is unremitting,* this occurs because as spirits are sent to the painful area they become disordered by the heat and as a result of this continuous transmission and disorder fever is constantly present, *moderating slightly during the day* because the soul (**85**) feels relieved after performing her internal function, and the spirits and humors are not so completely disordered, *but becoming more severe at night* because the catarrhal condition is exaggerated at night more than by day, resulting in an even greater transmission of spirits and greater disorder.

Profuse sweating and an unproductive cough occur when the trachea is compressed by an abscess of the breathing apparatus, thus producing an obstacle from which the cough results. At intervals there may be a false calm when they seem to have a trifling relief, but suddenly they begin to cough again *and the eyeballs protrude* from fumes pressing on the eyes which are transmitted to them because they have a common boundary with the breathing apparatus. *And there is redness at the angles of the eyes* because the stinging of the fumes produces an opening of the veins so that blood exudes and a red color predominates. *And there is constriction at the fingertips* (86), because of heat and dryness; along with this tendency of dryness to constrict *the fingers grow hot* from warm fumes transmitted to them *and especially to their tips* because heat has a motion from the center which becomes more powerful in the external parts. *And small abscesses form and disappear on the feet* because of the fumes transmitted to them, *and they suffer from loss of appetite,* either because there is loss of the spirits needed to stimulate the required virtue of the stomach or because of the humors becoming corrupt. There is a release of such corrupt fumes which appear at the mouth of the stomach giving rise to squeamishness and loathing, and because of these fumes *vesicles arise on the body* but they do not continue in this way, being first composed of wind, but *soon become filled with pus* and discharge a bloody matter (87).

These are the signs by which empyema is quickly recognized: the author has spoken above about the termination of abscesses and has defined the termination of putrid abscesses, but not of empyema. He therefore now introduces the subject of the termination of empyema, and mentions some signs by which we can investigate this subject. *Among the signs mentioned you shall note whether breathing is rapid,* that is, whether the action of inspiration and expiration is too rapid: this occurs from excessive heat and dryness, so that the air, when drawn into the body cannot produce much dilation of the lung because of the dryness, and what is lost in even one exchange cannot be recovered as time goes on. *Expectoration with a persistent cough:* by passage of matter through the trachea the breathing is interfered with and cough results, and because of this bubbling over of matter from heat some of it is continuously being released, as may be seen in a boiling pot. The breathing is constantly interfered with and the resulting cough is called persistent, not only because it does not disappear but because it is non-productive. *And even with expectoration the patient may become worse* because very often the parts are compressed from the struggle of bringing up phlegm, and compression of the abscess increases, causing a further loss of continuity and thus more pain.

Expect the abscess to break before the twentieth day, for by then the boiling matter is changed into sanies, *and then they ask for food,* because the corrupt fumes which produce squeamishness are no longer being produced, nor are those weakening spirits present which cause the appetite to fail. *When the fever subsides on the same day that the abscess breaks you may judge that the patient will recover:* he implies here that the rupture

of an abscess occurs at times from natural heat, at other times from accidental heat, and that from such accidental heat the man dies whereas through natural heat he recovers.

Moderate and well-formed stools are useful, because they announce a strong motility of the stomach, the organ which is the father of the family (88), and *well-formed,* that is, midway between solid and liquid. *And the purulent matter expectorated is whitish* because strong natural heat produces boiling and bleaching, *and light,* because of the continued absence of wind, *and uniform throughout,* that is, in continuity, because there is an absence of wind in the whole and in the part. When in the whole and in the part the natural action of heat is strong and uniform *and produces no effort* or pain, it becomes apparent that the matter is not really of a fiery nature, *and a mild cough* results because of the small amount of matter and its lack of fury, so that there is little furious matter *coming to the trachea* which might irritate and produce more coughing. *In this way they are quick to recover* because such discharges indicate the strength of the natural forces. *And others are close to recovery,* that is, there is a rapid termination of the illness in those whose *signs are closest* or most similar to the signs mentioned above.

There are those in whom fever does not subside even with the rupture of an abscess, because of strength of the accidental heat, *for without a sign, and stealthily, the matter returns after seeming to depart,* that is, it makes sport of nature, and destructive matter is seen to be retained even after the rupture of the abscess; indeed after that discharge there is a recirculation of the harmful matter and a new collection forms which is worse than the earlier one because it is now laid bare and open. *And they are afflicted with great thirst because of frequent eliminations* and *have no appetite* because of nauseating fumes. And the stools carried off are soft: such stools occur because of the strength of symptoms and lack of control over matter and therefore they verge on softness. *Later a livid color* develops because of mortification *or it may be livid* because of inflammation, *or mixed with phlegm* because of crudity, *and frothy* because all frothy matter with a color indicating heat is a sign of the fury of matter, while a color indicating cold implies the existence of indigestion and flatulence.

When these signs are protracted, you may certainly anticipate the death of some patients who have ineffective resources; *not all will die but others will remain alive* who have better and more effective resources, *and therefore the ending is difficult to predict* for the physician, because these are perplexing cases and the prognostic signs are hidden. *These signs must be uncovered by your discerning judgment,* that is, the signs must be carefully differentiated.

31. [*Prognostics XVIII*] *In cases of pneumonia and so forth:* the author intends to define the termination of the pneumonic abscess, the so-called "first born"

because derived from another abscess, as *in those cases of pneumonia with abscesses about the ears*, that is, either above or below the ears (**89**). *Such an abscess may develop* when matter from the primitive abscess is diverted to the superior parts and *putridity results*, for through matter boiling over, it is transformed into putridity, *and as this breaks through a fistula develops*, that is, there is a flow of sanies which escapes in this way. When matter appears through the fistula this continuing flow of sanies is regenerated daily and this indicates mortification of that part located in close proximity to the ear or just below it, or of other parts having a similar supply of veins, arteries, and nerves. The matter of an abscess collects in a point and because of the excessive sensitivity and rush of humors pain results. Many humors cross this area and run about, causing the part to become putrid. There is no dispersal from one member to another, but the flow is toward the surface parts, either continuous or contiguous, so that little by little the matter follows through one part and then another until a fistula develops.

Be very careful, O physician, that in your study you show diligence and *weigh matters according to these precepts*, which means that you should investigate them thoroughly. *If fever persists:* the author now lays down certain good and bad signs, and if the good are more weighty than the bad the patient will be restored to health. First he mentions the bad signs rather than the good: it is bad for fever to linger on because of a persistent abscess in the superficial parts: *pain remains undiminished* because of the rush of humors to this very sensitive place, *and expectoration causes discomfort* because the temperate humor is lacking. *If the stool* is not bilious, that is, not humid, this is a good sign because the discharge remains midway between liquid and solid, and is *not too loose because of mortification.* *If the urine is moderate* this may be a good sign or a bad one, *but if the sediment is not too thick*, that is, if such a sediment appears daily until the termination by crisis this is a good sign which declares the completion of the third digestion in the parts, and if the third digestion is good, so were the second and the first. *All these signs are beneficial*, as is also the easy action of inspiration and expiration.

You may anticipate future abscesses around the ear: because nature, now expulsive, waxes strong in the entire body including the brain, and if that matter is sufficiently potent it is driven to the brain by its own power, but the strong expulsive nature of the brain drives it below the ear. *Abscesses often arise here when there has been pain and heat in the hypochondria* so that when matter is collected in the lungs it gathers in the upper angles from which it is rushed to a point above the ear, and this being close to the brain may prove fatal (**90**). When the matter is collected in the inferior parts of the lung this indicates that the matter was cold, so that it is drawn to lower parts and is collected

below the ear, but because it does not come close to the brain it does not bring on death. *In cases of pneumonia the inferior hypochondria are without pain or heat:* but the superior hypochondria are painful and feverish as in the wings of the lung *and following these abscesses develop around the ear* because such abscesses are also warm.

32. *Abscesses and so forth:* termination of a pulmonic abscess may result from the transmission of black bile not only to the ears but also to the feet, the matter present in the lung being sent by an artery to the feet where it produces an abscess. *It is best when expectoration begins early*, for there is no better way for pneumonia to end than by the ejection of sputum, and it is an especially good sign when red sputum is changed into white by the power of nature. *In these signs you may find safety*, that is, even when the sputum ejected is not yet what it should be, being thick, globular, green or black. *Nor should the sediment in the urine be distrusted, although when an abscess develops in this organ great danger must be anticipated* because it spreads widely and may bring on death, or as happens in a number of cases, the matter is carried to the feet or to another member, and that member, being humid, becomes putrid and falls off (**91**). *But indeed if the abscess disappears*, being abducted to the superior parts, *but the fever does not abate*, this brings on death, *especially in those who are aged*, that is, who are greatly advanced in age, because older people *perish from pulmonic suppuration*, and since all this occurs in the presence of a cold humor they die because of the protracted nature of the illness. *Others indeed are more greatly affected by different types of suppuration*, such as youths with pleurisy, a disease in which everything becomes sharply localized at one point.

33. [*Prognostics XIX*] *In acute fevers and so forth:* the author now intends to consider a collection of matter which goes on to form an abscess in the kidneys; *this is attended by acute fever*, indicating the presence of acute matter which accompanies an acute fever. *If there is pain in the loins* then the matter causing this pain *ascends from the kidneys to the region above the diaphragm* where the heart lies; and the matter being warm and dry has the power of drying and dissolving, and by crossing from an ignoble to a noble part it sets up a pleurisy. *Nevertheless having examined these various signs*, do not be hasty in your judgment to predict death for the sufferer, but you must judge from the abundance or infrequency of signs, for if you see a preponderance of good signs do not predict death, on the other hand if more signs are unfavorable you may predict death.

If the bladder is painful because of the collection of matter to form an abscess in the bladder and so forth: the bladder is a cold organ, and therefore cannot suffer pain unless the matter is of a bilious nature *and hard*, that is, firm because of dryness (**92**). Thus if the matter is warm and dry, not warm and humid, and fevers are not extinguished readily because the matter does not turn into sanies or into a firm substance, *you may predict danger* because the matter is retained there and cannot be led off because of an obstruction; and with the power of drying this brings additional peril *which becomes intensified by a stricture of the intestinal tract,* for the rectum, at its beginning, has a common boundary with the bladder, and if an abscess occurs in the abdomen the rectum is compressed (**93**), thus preventing an exit to the superfluity of the first digestion and of the second.

If the urine appears to be full of pus, that is, very cloudy, *and of sediment,* and contains many humors, *the pain is lessened,* for with the cessation of the cause comes the cessation of the effect. *But if the urine does not* become cloudy with sediment *and the bladder does not become soft* and the abscess of the bladder is not turned into sanies, *and the fever persists, death will occur in the first period,* or more specifically on the seventh day, because both the stool and urine are being retained. *Another type occurs more often in the young between the ages of seven and twenty* because in these individuals, heat and humidity being very strong, there is constriction of the passages so that the humidity in solution cannot be led forth through the open pores but becomes concentrated in the bladder, collects there, and produces a new abscess. An abscess cannot develop in the genitals because they possess the most subtle humidity and are most efficient in destroying harmful humors. And especially is this true in young people because they possess frank humidity opposing the heat and have open passages through which harmful humors are dispersed.

SECTION THREE

34. [*Prognostics XX*] *Fevers come to an end and so forth:* here begins the third section which is devoted to the spiritual virtue, so that the signs considered here are related to the strength or weakness of this spiritual virtue. The author indicates that it is by fever that the spiritual virtue is injured most effectively, because in fact he has already told us in the preceding text that some illnesses terminate on the seventh day, others on the fourteenth, and still others on the twentieth, and that in every case the termination may result in death or recovery. But lest anyone should think that the end is preordained toward recovery rather than toward death, our author removes this idea by saying *fevers terminate* on the very same day *on which the sick die or recover.* The author is about to define the spiritual signs relating to the termination of fever and he first cites certain general signs by which one may anticipate a favorable or an unfavorable development in an illness.

Turning first to recovery he discusses *those fevers in which all the symptoms have been favorable,* that is, all signs which appear favor recovery, such as good bowel

movements and the like, so that *anticipation of evil* or fear of evil *does not persist in this case* or have any close association, for no sign of evil appears. If these favorable signs appear on the appointed day, *namely on the fourth,* the one truly appointed for this purpose, according to the four-day cycle; *or earlier,* that is, on the third day when this is the day appointed, then you may expect a favorable termination and the patient will recover. For instance, in a four-day cycle the signs may appear on the eleventh or fourteenth day, in a three-day cycle on the thirteenth, yet the patient will recover.

The author now defines the signs indicating that the disease will end badly, as when all evil signs make their appearance on the appointed critical day. If this occurs on the day appointed for the termination, namely on the fourth, then the illness will end badly, and he adds: *but in those in whom dangerous symptoms appear with no moderating signs by the fourth day,* this being the appointed day, or before that, by the third day, *then death will certainly occur.* Because such illnesses usually terminate on the critical days he now treats of these, calling *the first period,* "universal." "First" is evidently intended to relate to the number "twenty," for in this latter number is contained a period which may be universal or particular. This universal period contains six items, so that this first period of twenty days includes four, seven, eleven, fourteen, seventeen, and twenty, that is, *the first period ends on the fourth, the second on the seventh, the third on the eleventh, the fourth on the fourteenth, the fifth on the seventeenth, and the sixth on the twentieth:* this progression by fours in acute illnesses runs over to the twentieth day. Following this first twenty, you may proceed in similar fashion to the twentieth twenty (**94**).

But these periods cannot be counted by whole days and so forth: here Hippocrates tacitly replies to his opponents. For it may be asked why the fourteenth and twenty-fourth days are judged critical because these are even numbers, and according to what he says in the *Aphorisms,* only odd numbers are to be regarded as having the correct proportion and disposition for a crisis. And because "septimana," or week, is so called from "septimo," or seventh, and three weeks make twenty-one days, why then do three weeks terminate within a period of twenty days? To this, the author replies that *these periods are not to be counted by whole days,* that is, by a complement, for "in" and "completum" are two parts of the word "incompletum," *and in fact neither the year nor the months are to be counted in whole numbers,* but we must count them by an odd or incomplete number analogous to their form, just as we say *three weeks end in a period of twenty days,* so it is permissible to say that a year ends within a period of 365 days, and a month ends within a period of twenty-nine or thirty days, and we may speak in a similar way about other things.

Nevertheless, according to the correct reckoning of

the astronomers, a year is the period of time during which the sun clearly traverses the entire zodiac. In this period are 365 days and six hours, and for this reason a leap year occurs every fourth year, six hours or a quarter of a day being added every year so that in three years eighteen are added. By the fourth year, the six hours added to the eighteen complete an entire day, whence that year is called a leap year, containing one complementary day. A month is a period of twenty-nine days and twelve hours in which period the moon clearly traverses its entire zodiac. Now just as at one time the entire year, and at another time the month, are counted by a whole number of days, so must the week also be counted by a whole number of days. But the period of a week actually is six days and sixteen hours, in which interval nature executes three of its motions. Therefore, three times six makes eighteen, three times sixteen makes forty-eight hours which, divided by two, makes two days, which added to the eighteen make twenty, and thus three weeks terminate in a period of twenty days (95).

From this, or rather *following this* argument, *there is good reason for extending the first*, or so-called universal, *period, thus the termination of the abscess may occur on the twentieth day, secondly on the fortieth and thirdly on the sixtieth*. It seems, however, that the author contradicts himself here, for in the *Aphorisms* at the section beginning *Acute illnesses and so forth* Hippocrates explained to us what he understood about acute illnesses not complicated by abscesses (96), while here he is talking about acute disease complicated by abscesses; or we may say that he was there speaking about continuous, acute diseases such as the continuous tertian and the like, whereas here he is discussing protracted, non-acute diseases, such as the continuous quartan and other diseases whose termination may be postponed until the sixtieth day.

35. *In certain diseases and so forth:* our author earlier considered the various terminations of abscesses and stated that some terminate on the twentieth day, others on the fortieth, and still others on the sixtieth. Now he discusses certain illnesses in which the termination is further delayed, and these may be recognized by the fact that the prognostic signs are obscure. Moreover, this delay is related to the remission of heat, the weakness of nature, the crudity of waste matter and the impaction of such matter, all of which cause the disease to be protracted. He therefore adds *in those diseases*, or illnesses, *in which the prognostic sign of recovery is late in arriving*, that is, the sign of recovery, *the signs of the onset of the disease are hidden, and it is difficult to decide just when the disease began*, for what we consider the point of increase of the disease may really be the true beginning, and so in similar cases, no clear signs of death or life appear. *One should therefore study attentively* whether a specific ailment ought to terminate by a three- or four-day cycle, and observe whether nature is moved on the third or

fourth day. From what you can observe of the prognostic signs, you may judge of the final event, and whether the illness will terminate by a three- or four-day cycle. *In those with a four-day cycle*, once the progression has been discovered, *be very attentive, because if you watch carefully, you will hardly ever fail, and the disease will end on a day which is related to the number four, and in this manner*, we see the usefulness of determining whether the disease will end by way of fours.

Hippocrates said earlier that if at the outset the prognostic signs are hidden the termination will be delayed. Now he adds that *it is easier to recognize the diseases which will end briefly*, when the prognostic signs are clear from the onset, *for their differences are very obvious*, but before the illness ends in recovery the physician may erroneously predict a calamity. Therefore, the author considers certain prognostic signs by which a correct determination of future life or death can be made, saying that *those who will survive breathe easily*, because from this the strength of the respiratory virtue can be observed, *and suffer no pain* nor any sign of its presence, *and sleep naturally at night*, because sleep indicates an excellent disposition of the brain and its membranes, *so that all these signs* are favorable as enumerated, and furthermore the sick man has an appetite for food and has good control of himself, so that all together these signs point to recovery.

Now, the author considers the prognostic signs of future death, saying *those who are about to die have labored breathing*, that is, rapid respiration and expiration, which indicate inflammation of the respiratory organs, *a confused mind*, the mind being confused because of disturbance of the humors, and *constant wakefulness*, from pain or dryness of the brain, *and these are heralds of calamity*, that is, are warnings of death as when, for example, the patient is not in control of himself, and so forth. But because he said above that if good signs begin with the onset of the illness, they give notice of recovery, and their absence, on the contrary, of death, lest any general principle of immunity be implied he removes this idea by adding *you must therefore pay close attention to the progress of every disease until the crisis*, because if favorable signs appear at the onset, one must observe whether they continue in this manner until the peak of the illness, for the good signs may change to bad, and you must now prognosticate as to future life or death. *One must be careful in applying what has been pointed out above with regard to pregnant or non-pregnant women;* if all signs of evil persist until the peak of the illness the crisis will confirm these by announcing death.

36. [*Prognostics XXI*] *If there is pain in the head, and so forth:* the author is about to prognosticate concerning abscesses of the brain, because before an abscess develops in the dura mater there is acute pain, and when it exists in the pia mater the pain is more

acute; and when in the substance of the brain the pain is most severe (**97**). Therefore he says: *if the pain in the head is very severe* this indicates that a collection of pus is being formed in the substance of the brain, and *if fever is present* this signifies the presence of bilious matter in the head by the acuteness of which the brain—from which all other members are said to take their origin—is dissolved and death ensues (**98**). *And if a deadly sign appears* this leads to a mood of apprehension and mental alienation and *death comes on rapidly*; but if no evil sign appears, that is, if there are none of the unfavorable signs previously mentioned by Hippocrates, *and the pain continues as long as the twentieth day*, it may be inferred that nature is of sufficient strength to sustain the pain, however severe, *and if fever continues* this implies that the matter did not collect to form an abscess in the brain but was diverted by the strength of nature to a lower member where it will terminate in an abscess. Nature, being very active in discovering new passages, takes the matter not yet gathered to form an abscess and evacuates it through a nosebleed.

Indeed, he says *you may expect hemorrhage from the nose or an abscess in the lower extremities; but if the pain persists, you will hope for such a hemorrhage from the nose or an abscess,* because this signifies that the matter did not become congealed to form an abscess, but will be evacuated by a flux of blood, and it is *most preferable* that the matter be so expelled by a flow of blood. *When pain persists in the forehead and temples* this indicates that the matter is close to the venules of the nose, and can be evacuated more quickly this way than through formation of another abscess. The author lays down the signs through which abscesses of the brain can most effectively be diagnosed, and shows that depending upon the patient's age, the abscess will terminate through a nasal hemorrhage or by formation of another abscess, adding that you will hope for a flow of blood, *especially in those who are under thirty-five* and younger, that is, in youths in whom the vigor of nature is great and the heat acute. Indeed, you will look for *an abscess in those who are older*, as in the aged in whom strength is reduced and heat lost, so that nature, having become less effective, takes matter from noble to ignoble organs, and thus a termination occurs by an acute abscess forming in the lower parts.

37. [*Prognostics XXII*] *Acute pain in the ear and so forth*: the author at this point intends to prognosticate about abscesses around the ear. Pain may develop in the area, at times from a single quality such as dissolving heat, constricting cold, loosening humidity and destructive dryness. At other times, a quality combines with a humor to form an abscess; because some matter continuously develops a crust and the warm humor produces a boiling over; from this boiling over a resolution occurs; the spirits are in a constant state of disorder and a continuous fever lingers on. But if the abscess is derived from a cold humor the fever will be continuous though not severe, whereas when derived from a warm humor the fever will be continuous, severe, and accompanied by acute pain around the ears. Therefore, he speaks of *severe pain around the ear*, by which we can recognize the presence of acute matter heated to boiling. *A continuation of such signs is serious, and you must expect delirium and death:* for the matter, being very hot and near the brain, tears apart the substance of the brain by its sharpness and thus brings on death. By corrupting and disturbing the spirit, it causes alienation, *and such a case is grave and dangerous* because of that abscess, and all these people die—some earlier, some later.

You must therefore be careful, or rather, it is to your advantage, O physician, *to scan all signs* of abscesses, and *to scrutinize the symptoms from the very first day, because young people who are attacked*, or who are affected by this disease, *perish on the seventh day or even earlier*, that is, on the fifth. For youths, from the nature of their complexion and age, are hot and dry and this type of abscess is derived from extremely hot and dry matter, so that the condition becomes doubly dangerous from the action of heat, the complexion and age, with the result that nature, exhausted by the sharpness of the matter, succumbs. *Older people die much later* from this kind of abscess because from age and complexion they are cold, so that even the matter cannot be rarified and dispersed because of the weakness of the heat; nevertheless it is clear that the development of such matter indicates the early approach of death (**99**). *Because fever and delirium attack them less violently than young people* because of diminished heat and the lessened virulence of the matter the disease drags on, *but their ears*, that is of the older people, *break open and discharge*, that is, *purulent matter is evacuated in persons of advanced age*, because their nature being weakened from the peculiarity of age is unable to cleanse itself perfectly of the pus through formation of sanies. As a result, the disease *relapses and intermits* over a long period of time. *Young people die before suppuration can begin* from the excessive acuteness and fury of the matter. For nature, even in its prime, is not able to withstand the acuteness of this abscess. *But if pus should form and break through,* that is, in youths, *and other favorable symptoms* appear, and the patient's mind is not disturbed, but he is rather in good control of himself, *you may hope that this patient will live*, that is, you may hope for a recovery, *for the matter* by the effort of nature has been converted into sanies and eliminated.

38. [*Prognostics XXIII*] *Abscess in the throat and so forth:* the author is concerned here with abscesses of the throat which have their origin in the pharynx, rather than with quinsy, as some think. In fact, this form of abscess arises from a catarrh, when humors flowing from the head to the throat suddenly attack the pharynx or "antimeron," and through the injurious action of heat crusts develop and thus an abscess is formed.

And therefore Hippocrates says, *an abscess in the throat accompanied by acute fever is very bad,* for as a result the action of inspiration and expiration and the swallowing of food and drink are impeded. *If other unfavorable signs develop among those already mentioned* such as insanity or some other, the patient *will die.*

39. *Quinsy and so forth:* here the author deals with abscesses which occur within the isthmus of the throat, namely in a certain follicle, which is located between the two principal parts, namely between the trachea and the esophagus. Different terms are assigned to these abscesses according to various locations of the matter. If the entire matter is collected within the isthmus the abscess is called "quinsy," if entirely outside, "squinancia," if partly within and partly without, "sinancia." Although *all of these are very dangerous,* quinsy is the most dangerous of all, and it is impossible to free anyone from this condition unless the matter can be diverted to the superior parts, for so long as the matter lies entirely within the isthmus it constricts the esophagus and blocks access to food and drink. The trachea is also compressed and by this constriction inspiration and expiration are impeded, and this is followed by sudden choking. Sinancia is not quite so dangerous, and it is possible to free a patient from it unless the matter occupies a position deeply within the isthmus, and the matter remaining on the surface seeks to unite with matter in the interior parts. All are freed from squinantia unless the matter is diverted internally.

Therefore he states that quinsy is the worst and most rapidly fatal: among various abscesses which are accompanied by fever none is more dangerous and more deadly than this because a wasting and inflammation of the organ of breathing develops from the high fever with the result that there is a pressing need for fresh air which must be drawn in to cool off the innate distemper. However, such intake of air cannot occur, because the abscess present in the isthmus and trachea results in a constriction, nor can fumes be exhaled and thus choking results. *And there is nothing visible in the throat,* thus indicating that the matter is almost entirely collected in the interior parts, *nor does it spread to the neck with redness and swelling,* because all the matter is internal, *but as the severe pain persists* the fierceness of the matter can be estimated. Then follows *orthopnea,* or breathing in the upright position, for with the matter accumulating in the isthmus the trachea is compressed so that free inspiration and expiration cannot continue properly and thus the free intake of air and the free exhalation of fumes are impeded, and if the latter are diverted to the neck there results a great constriction of the trachea and choking results. *In severe cases the patient may suffocate on the first, second, third, or fourth day:* he thus lays down the final point beyond which they cannot go, and to which in fact they seldom if ever arrive.

Now, he considers in the same way the second variety, called sinancia, saying *another variety occurs with swelling and redness of the throat* because the matter may be collected partly inwardly and partly outwardly. *This is also deadly, but not so rapidly* as the aforementioned, because destruction is delayed longer and life continues for a longer period.

He then discusses the third variety, saying that *the third type occurs when the neck and throat both become very red, and is much more protracted than the previous types,* that is, it lasts for a much longer time. *And unless the swelling turns inwards,* by which he means that the matter is abducted to the interior, *all hope of recovery is not lost,* that is, there is some hope for future recovery. *But if the disease has remained concealed,* that is, if it appeared quite suddenly *yet not on the critical day itself,* this indicates that the matter was turned inwards by artificial means, *and that it was not the developing of another abscess* that caused the swelling to be diverted elsewhere. By this he implies that the matter was not diverted to form another abscess in the interior parts; *nor is there any lasting discharge of pus* which shows that the matter was not reduced to sanies by the action of heat and can by no means be evacuated. *Rather it may disappear gradually* showing that the matter is being destroyed little by little; *and there may be relief of pain so that the patient becomes quiet,* for when the matter is entirely diverted into the interior parts and is absorbed by the very substance of the individual he seems to be relieved, yet when the matter approaches the organs of breathing it again induces choking and *this may imply that death or a recurrence of distress is at hand.* But at times there is not enough matter to induce choking, and the virtue of the organs of breathing being strong, when the matter does arrive, they repel it and send it back to its original location where, not being entirely innocuous it may bring on a relapse.

It is good if the swelling becomes red and protrudes outward because this indicates a discharge of matter to the exterior, *for if the abscess remains internal, the matter of the abscess may extend to the lungs, and a purulent condition may develop there* by the action of heat, *with a recurrence of delirium,* because from such putrid matter putrid fumes are released which, arriving at the brain destroy its substance and bring on madness.

40. *The uvula being red and swollen and so forth:* the author has prognosticated above concerning abscesses of the throat, now he intends to prognosticate about abscesses of the uvula, a certain member which hangs from the palate in a manner resembling the nipple of the breasts. It is also called "uva" because of its resemblance to a bunch of grapes, the part above being broad and continuous with the palate, but coming to a sharp point below. The upper part is contained in a large aperture, the lower in a small. Now this member is appointed by nature to carry off the superfluities of the brain, and its lower part is contained in a

small aperture so that when the superfluities arrive there they are gradually expelled by coughing. If the aperture were too large, the humor dripping down suddenly in large quantities on the organs of respiration would cause suffocation. Or the uvula was placed there by nature to purify the inspired air, for if dusty air is inhaled it is cleansed because the dust adheres to the substance of that member and being later mixed with sputum is thrown off in the expectoration. Moreover, this organ contains much blood, and occasionally an abscess develops causing the uvula to become swollen with sharp and localized pain. The pain is localized when phlegm collects in a natural manner and the uvula is only partly swollen, the pain becoming more widespread as the organ develops a whitish color. At other times bile predominates and then the organ is saffron-colored or yellow, and the pain piercing; when black bile predominates it assumes an earthy color and the pain, being more generalized, is felt little or not at all.

Hippocrates suggests two methods of treatment: at the appropriate time the golden cautery can be applied, followed by drying medications, or it can be cured by incision (**100**). But because the danger of suffocation is great the patient should first be given a general purgation, then an opiate should be administered before the incision is made at a time considered favorable. In this way the danger of suffocation is diminished. But he adds, if the weather is catarrhal and *the uvula is swollen and red*, thus indicating the presence of bloody matter, *to cut with the knife* is very dangerous because sanies follows in a continuous flow from the uvula, and the perforated area is unable to form a scar so long as the humors which flow down are changed into sanies. The patient thus becomes empyemic, that is, from the excretion of purulent sanies, an empyema develops which changes into a phthisis (**101**). *Or excessive hemorrhage continues* producing a bloody swelling, so that you should try other methods, such as the cautery or the application of drying medications. *But if you cannot avoid an incision and the uvula becomes even larger and more livid*, this enlargement implies that the matter is not being consumed and the lividity indicates mortification, *and the upper part adhering to the palate is thinned out*, thus indicating that the heavier matter has settled in the lower part, *then incise, but first prepare the entire body* by purges as previously mentioned, *and see that the weather is favorable*, that is, not catarrhal, when fluxes occur, *and there is no danger of suffocation*.

And because this kind of abscess is accompanied by fever, he adds that *if the fever gradually lessens* this implies that some small part of the matter is being consumed; *but if there is no sign of the end of the illness, and no disappearance of the fever on the critical day*, this indicates that the matter has not been consumed and is being collected in large quantity, then *you may anticipate a relapse*, but because the heat is being stifled

the fever gradually beomes lighter. A bit later on a severe inflammation of the matter brings on repletion of the abscess and a recurrence of the previous symptoms.

Having outlined the cure of abscess of the uvula and the signs by which a recurrence may be recognized, he now considers the method of termination, whether or not this is to occur through the formation of another abscess, or through abscesses of the joints. For nature being earlier too weak to bring about a complete crisis does as much as it can, and transports matter from the noble to ignoble parts, and especially to those members where the attractive virtue is vigorous because of motion, namely the articulations and the joints (**102**). In these cases, therefore, while the matter is being covered over through the action of heat a crust develops on the abscess, and thus the abscess of the uvula comes to an end.

[*Prognostics XXIV*] He then says *in those cases where fever lingers on* this signifies that matter is still present, around which heat maintains a continuous boiling, causing a persistent fever. *Nor are these abscesses generated with distress to the patient*: this signifies that the matter is crude and cold, so that the sick man is not greatly troubled, *nor is the uvula very painful*, thus signifying that the matter is crude and concentrated, so that heat, maintaining a minimum of boiling, induces only a slight loss of continuity. *You may anticipate abscesses and swellings, especially in the lower* extremities, from weightiness which causes matter to move downward. *But if the fever continues* beyond the twentieth day, counting from the onset of fever, this occurs because the matter is highly concentrated and requires a long time for its digestion.

Now the author informs us how these abscesses terminate at different ages, and in what ages they are less apt to occur. Referring to these very abscesses of the joints of the lower extremities, he says *they are less apt to occur in persons below forty-five years of age* (**103**) because in them heat is so strong that by its action the matter is destroyed or reduced to sanies, or by the vigor of nature the matter is entirely transferred to other parts and fever terminates immediately. But in *those whose age is greater*, that is, in the elderly, in whom an abscess of this type arises as a sequel, and there is a persistence of fever, indeed this occurs in the aged because in them nature is truly weak, and the heat being mild, many superfluities are generated which augment the matter of the disease, so that as a result of overly weak nature, part of the matter is permitted to be sent to the joints of the bones where it is collected to form an abscess. The part which remains is nevertheless sufficient to induce fever, which thus lingers on.

41. *Continuous fevers and so forth*: Hippocrates intends to prognosticate about various paroxysms in disease (**104**). Paroxysm means an exacerbation and may be orderly or disorderly, an orderly paroxysm

being one which flares up regularly and seizes the patient, as in a tertian with three days elapsing from one seizure to another. A disorderly paroxysm is so called because not being in accordance with the rule of three it may attack now every third day, now every fourth, fifth, and so forth. This implies the control of diverse humors, for at one time it may be bile which putrifies and produces its action, at other times it may be phlegm or black bile. Therefore he says *if fevers are unusually erratic*, that is, if they are spoken of as wandering or roving, *you may look for a quartan derived from black bile*, for this humor, being more concentrated than the others, causes harm later than the other humors. Bile is another humor which by its nature resists being changed into pus and requires a long time for its digestion, so that after other humors are destroyed this erratic one is changed into a quartan, or rather the bile, having become inflamed by the heat, produces a quartan. *This is more likely to occur in autumn:* for then the humors derived from black bile are generated more actively because of the weather's harshness, *and especially among those persons* previously mentioned, namely, old people, *and just as abscesses arise in those who have passed thirty-five, so do quartans attack those who are older*, because the combination of cold and dryness prevails in all older people.

42. *Abscesses and so forth:* in the last section Hippocrates defined certain general rules about abscesses, saying *all abscesses are more apt* to form in the winter, that is, all varieties of abscesses are then more prevalent *than in other seasons*. This universal sign, "all," refers here to various classes of individuals, and not to individuals of a single class. Now the sanguine and biliary abscesses are nevertheless seen clearly to react in a manner contrary to this opinion, for bile is generated in large quantity by the liver in summer, and is then superabundant, so that the bilious abscess ought to occur more often in summer than in winter. To which we reply that in summer, no matter how much bile is generated, it cannot coalesce in one place or become concentrated, because the air's heat, by opening the pores causes the bile to become dissolved in fumes and to evaporate. In winter on the other hand, no matter how small the quantity of bile generated the pores are constricted by the excessive cold, and the retained bilious superfluities having a motion of their own toward the center are concentrated in one place and being covered by a crust become revealed as an abscess. Nor does this occur in any random part of the body, but primarily in the organs of respiration, because it is to that part that many cold and weak superfluities are sent. Although in autumn much black bile is generated, because of nearness to summer heat is still retained in the air so that the pores being open the fumes evaporate, but this does not happen in winter. The sanguine abscess is more common in winter because of the many fumes generated which mix with the blood itself than it is in the spring when pure blood is generated. From another point of view an abscess may be considered primary or secondary, the latter being derived from another abscess, just as we have spoken about the abscess around the ear being secondary to pneumonia.

All secondary abscesses occur more frequently in winter than in other seasons because many superfluities are then generated, and these being first collected in one place are later transmitted by their own weight to other parts and collected into abscesses. *And they die more frequently* because of the excess of matter, *but others get well and do not relapse:* some wish to explain that nature is then strong, so that later the abscess is changed into sanies and the matter entirely evacuated, and the member remaining strong, prevents the free flow of matter so that no relapse occurs. On the other hand at other seasons when the members are weakened the matter already purified offers an obstacle to the flow of the humor, indeed there may be a reversal of the flow. Or from another point of view, in summer because of dryness, the matter of an abscess is condensed so that it is almost destroyed by the heat, but a bit later, reactivating itself, it goes back into solution and thus the abscess changes its state back and forth. But in winter the air is cold, and heat, by whose action the matter is changed into sanies is excluded, and once the matter is led off by the strength of nature there is no remission (**105**).

In those who have fever and so forth: having laid down the signs of the various types of abscesses, he now considers the signs derived from fever by which you may estimate the termination of various diseases, especially the intermittent, as can also be done for the tertian through the vomitus. And he adds *in those who have fevers which are not fatal:* fevers which are not fatal are called intermittent with respect to their long continuation and from the fact that nature never succumbs to the virulence of the disease. Or they are described as not deadly because no prognostic sign of death seems to appear, or because Hippocrates is not really referring to tertian fever, his attention being directed only to acute diseases.

Concerning these acute diseases he now prognosticates, for a tertian may be true or false. The true tertian is one in which all the particulars, or at least most of them, are in accord with the properties of natural matter; the false is one in which all the particulars, or most of them, are not in accord with the properties of natural matter; rather it arises from abnormal matter. Here, therefore, when he speaks of the tertian he does not generalize, but refers to the acute type of the disease which is quickly fatal unless it becomes intermittent. There is a short-lived type of the disease in which, when the individual's strength has been reduced by exertion, nature may be restored by a day of rest. It is short-lived because being made of matter which is warm and dry, the matter is rarified by this heat and dryness, and once rarified is quickly destroyed, whence in the *Aphorisms* (106) it is concluded that a true tertian should come to a crisis within seven periods at the latest.

If there is complaint of pain in the head this indicates the presence of bilious matter which, being light, is controlled by heat and easily dissolved into fumes which seek the brain and thus induce pain in the brain with loss of continuity. *And patients think that they see flies before their eyes*, for matter coming to rest at the mouth of the stomach has direct access and free progress to the upper parts and is made ready for digestion by the heat increasing within. It is then dissolved into many fumes which, being sent to the anterior cell of the brain (107), discolor the spirit of sight so that even if an object is round, it assumes this appearance, and if subtle and elongated, objects appear as small bodies, and this is as it should be. *But things appear dark*, this indicates greater action of heat on matter, so that when it is dissolved into fumes by the action of heat, it becomes burned and blackened, and thus the spirit of sight is discolored so that everything appears to the patient as black in color, and this he considers a very distinctive sign.

And if the pain travels to the vital organs—the organs of breathing are called vital—and then radiates almost to the mouth of the stomach, because of the great overheating which results, the organs of respiration are compressed and their distress is made evident by these signs: *you may expect a vomiting of reddish bile*, he adds this as a distinctive sign; and *if cold*, that is, if a chill *is present* this means that the chill arises from warm matter arriving at the mouth of the stomach which stings and burns and produces a chill. *And if cold is felt in the hypochondria* this indicates that when matter is abducted to the mouth of the stomach by its presence the lower hypochondria become heated; conversely, by its absence they become cold.

A certain and sudden vomiting may be expected: he now adds with certainty that *if the patient has taken anything by mouth he will very soon reject it*, for if there is matter present at the mouth of the stomach because of the overpowering ebullition produced by heat foods are expelled to the exterior.

The author now considers signs by which an early or late crisis may be diagnosed, considering first *those in whom head pains begin with the onset of fever:* this indicates an aptitude of the matter for being digested, because at the onset matter can easily be dissolved by the action of heat. *In the fourth and fifth day the pain increases*, thus indicating an increase of fever; the peak of the illness now follows and on the seventh day they escape from danger, because nature being sufficiently powerful to digest the matter expels it, and such a crisis leads to recovery. *But in those cases where the pain does not appear until the third day* this indicates that the matter is less under the control of the heat,

and increases until the fifth or seventh, he is here referring to the pain, then *it will end on the ninth or eleventh*, for if the pain increases to the fourth, it will end on the ninth; if it increases to the seventh, it will end on the eleventh, although the crisis itself may come later. Then he adds, *it may indeed happen* that the pain does not begin *until the fifth day*, thus indicating that the matter is not prepared for digestion in those *whose urine remains unchanged*, that is, in whom both urine and sediment are alike of reddish color. This indicates crudity of matter and a longer duration of the illness; or if a white, uniform sediment persists at the base, then the peak of the illness will be delayed, *but they will be freed on the fourteenth day*, that is, the crisis leads them to recovery. Therefore, it is necessary to go beyond the eleventh day if we are dealing with a four-day cycle.

Now what we have stated about tertians applies equally to men and women: he is referring not only to the event itself, but to the consequences. *In children* or in youths *the fevers are more protracted:* this is so with regard to a true tertian as it is in regard to a synocha and similar conditions. *Indeed in true tertians*, in which all signs conform with the property of matter, it is because they are warm and dry that all the details, or at least most of them, seem to accord with the properties of matter.

The author considered above the signs of the termination of fever by vomitus. Now he considers signs of impending hemorrhage, because at times blood putrifies in the lower veins beneath the hypochondria whence, by the strength of nature, the bloody matter is expelled upward to the superior parts and, by breaking the venules of the nose this blood is evacuated by a sudden flow. He says, therefore, *in those fevers accompanied by pain in the head*, this sign indicates the presence in the brain of humor and wind which by extending the meninges produce pain. *But if there are no black spots appearing before the eyes* this indicates the absence of inflamed bilious humor or black bile required to produce a resolution through vomitus; *but rather bright spots*, this signifies that the matter would be sanguineous, so that the dissolved fume exhibits bodies with a similar color. *And they have spasms under the right and left hypochondria*, that is, there are spasms indicating that bloody matter is being expelled to the superior parts thus causing the veins to become extended, *but the hypochondria are free of pain*, thus indicating that the bloody matter was not being collected to form an abscess, because then, being weighty, it could not have ascended to the superior parts. *In these cases there will be a hemorrhage from the nose as previously indicated.*

43. *Convulsions and so forth:* the author prognosticates about convulsions, indicating at what ages they are especially apt to occur. Convulsions occur either from an extension or contraction of the nerves or ten-

dons of the entire body, or from repletion, inanition or the presence of cold. The repleted nerves are contracted in length and drawn apart in width, thus producing convulsions, Again when exsiccated they dry out and then contract, convulsions later resulting from inanition. Again cold, having a motion toward the center and producing a shortening, contracts and shortens the part, so that convulsions may result from cold. Certain writings assign convulsions to repletion, saying *convulsions with fever occur in children* (108), that is, from the acuteness of the febrile heat. When the excessive humidity which abounds in children is dissolved by heat it fills the nerves and produces spasm from repletion, *especially if they are constipated* because this indicates retention of superfluities and a great sense of fullness; and they are sleepless because of great pain induced by fullness and cramps; *and they are frightened* because of diverse imaginings brought to the brain by the superabundant humors; *and they scream out* because of the excess of humor enclosed in the brain, part of which being sent to the eyes induces tears; *and they change color* according to the domination of various humors, *so that they become yellowish* from an excess of bile, *or reddish* from an excess of blood *or lead-colored* from an excess of black bile, *or almost greenish* because of a very severe inflammation.

Convulsions occur in children until they are seven, during which period their substantial humidity is great. But even in children this excessive humidity is apt to become dissolved and consumed by fever so that with loss of the customary humidity the nerves become desiccated, and once dried out, become contracted. Even abdominal constipation may result from this intensity of dryness which produces desiccated fecal matter. Presently wakefulness develops and nightmares, arising from the sharp, devouring heat and fever. It is not to be wondered at that they are frightened, because they carry within themselves the reason for fear. They weep because the natural humidity of the brain is dissolved, and when this is dissolved into humors by the action of heat the humors drip down and pass through the eyes producing tears.

Change of color arises from a variety of reactions to heat so that when bile is dissolved there develops a light yellow color, with blood a red color, with black bile a leaden-gray color, and when indeed there is an evil inflammation of humors a green color develops. All this occurs in children until they are seven, or as long as their humidity makes them prone to dissolution and wasting. *In older children,* that is, in *youths, convulsions do not occur* from inanition, nor *in fevers unless accompanied by severe symptoms such as delirium,* because in youths there is a much more compact humidity which can be consumed only by great heat and dryness, so that in these persons spasm from inanition does not occur.

44. At the end of his work the author warns the physician, charging him not to be negligent of prognostic signs, whether they indicate future death or recovery, for praise surely follows from the latter when he restores to health the sick man whom the fear of death prods on, or whom persistent pain tortures. From the former he also acquires fame (109) when he properly assigns a fatal prognosis to a man who is about to die. One should be attentive to the prognostic signs relating to the qualities of various ages. Compare the strength of the sick man with the strength of his illness, noting the signs of good and of evil. He adds *it is to your interest,* that is, to your advantage to be attentive, O physician, so that with much study you can *predict either death or recovery in children and youths in any sickness whatsoever,* but above all, *do not show yourself negligent.*

The author warns us that in any illness, whether brief or lengthy, whether serious or trivial, the physician must not appear negligent, but should be certain of the signs of life and death. *He is honored who can predict with certainty the recovery or death of a patient in acute or chronic diseases and can interpret the symptoms,* that is, he can distinguish the various signs, subject them to sound reason, and assess them in the manner already indicated. *You must be familiar with all the signs in urine and sputum:* for without doubt through the former you can recognize the disposition of the liver and urinary passages, through the sputum the condition of the respiratory organs. *And this is my teaching on acute diseases,* that these predictions be looked for in acute diseases.

Having defined the signs to be looked for in acute illnesses, he now discusses the signs which should be looked for in intermittent fevers, and even *long protracted epidemic diseases, such as cancer and others which linger on indefinitely* (110), and he indicated the special points to be looked for, saying *you must study the character of the prevalent diseases,* that is, the various stages of the current diseases, including their onset, development, peak, and decline, so that you will know how to apply suitable methods of cure. Lest anyone suppose that diseases arise in the same manner in one season of the year as in others, he says that *while all diseases may arise in every season of the year,* the word "all" is used here to comprehend classes of individual cases and not individual cases of a single class, and he is really speaking of all illnesses accompanied by pain. *And yet certain diseases are more frequent at various times of the year,* so that the tertian is more frequent in the summer, the quartan in autumn, and the quotidian in winter. He warns us that the physician must persist in studying the signs, saying *bad signs are always dangerous while good signs, on the other hand, are encouraging,* that is, those which appear good should be so considered, even though differing somewhat from signs in the usual course of the disease, and therefore they should be considered good, or at least not necessarily harmful.

To persuade us of his teachings he acknowledges that he has had experience in three parts of the world, adding that *these signs exist exactly as we have described them in Ethiopia, the northern regions and in the west,* that is to say, in Spain. *We are all well trained, nor should despair seize you because more often than you expect the sequence of signs will prove favorable to you,* that is, the sequence *will develop favorably as we have learned through many sleepless nights.* And because Hippocrates as a prophetic spirit (**111**) was able to anticipate the pseudo-physicians of the future and was concerned lest the true physician adhere to their false teachings, he dismisses us with the following precepts, enjoining us *not to search for other concepts of disease* or alien doctrines, *or even to search for other diseases* or signs of disease *because all diseases terminate in accordance with our enumeration,* that is, by three and fours, so that if you know the method already defined in our own precepts, then, O physician! you shall have acquired all the necessary knowledge through a study of my teachings.

COMMENTARY

1. References to the special significance and virtue of the number three are frequent in ancient and medieval science and medicine (see Lynn Thorndike, *A History of Magic and Experimental Science during the first Thirteen Centuries of our Era* [London, 1923] 1: p. 808), and this number also had an understandable appeal for medieval physicians. Typical citations in Maurus' writings include:

"Tocius humani corporis machina triplicis participatione qualitatis, tripliciter existens est variabilis, secundo nature sedulus inquisitor tripplicem signorum investigat seriem, eius dispositionem tripliciter reserantem, scilicet signa sumpta a forma corporis, ex actionibus eius et ex superfluitatibus" (*Commentarium in De Pulsibus Philareti* [BN 18499 164vA]).

"Materia Ipocratis in [h]oc opere est triplex, humani corporis alteratio que fit a naturalibus, non naturalibus et ab his que sunt contra naturam" (*Commentarium in Aphorismos* [CS 4: p. 514]).

Tribus namque incommodis subiacet corpus humanum, namque fluxui, alterationi et corruptioni. (*Regulae Urinarum* [CS 3: p. 2]). The same sentence appears in the *Commentarium in Aphorismos* [CS 4: p. 515] and see 1.25 ff. of our text.

2. In the absence of an organized *collegium*, individual masters competed actively for pupils, and living quarters as well as instruction were often provided at the master's house (H. P. Bayon, "Masters of Salerno and the Origins of Professional Medical Practice," *Science, Medicine and History: Essays in Honor of Charles Singer* [London, 1953]). The extent of professional rivalry can be guessed at from a sarcastic quip about the "deep and searching knowledge of a colleague" (Corner, *Anatomical Texts*, p. 60). Glosses were prepared or improvised by the master for the lemmata of the text being read, and these were then copied by students to be committed to memory. Because of this practice, versions of these *reportata* or *recollecta* vary greatly in reliability. Although master-pupil relationships may have been close, the pure altruism expressed in the following remarks of Master Salernus is open to question:

"Duplici me causa cogente, socii dilectissimi hoc opus instruere summo opere desudavi. Prima causa fuit finis utilitatis, secunda finis honestatis. Utile et enim est turba sociorum decorari, honestum est eorum utilitate clarescere. Communi ergo utilitati deserviens hic negotium breviter et utiliter componere non recusavi" (*CS* 5: p. 201).

Gilles de Corbeil speaks in the same vein:

"Sociis nostris domesticae fidei quorum gratia hoc opus suscepimus huius novae institutionis primicias offerimus . . . Ut mediocritate servata scholarium nostrorum qui doctrinae nostrae edulio cibantur, intelligentiae serviamus . . . Ut scholarium nostrorum eruditioni consuleremus et communi utilitati inserviremus" (C. Vieillard, *L'Urologie*, pp. 191–192).

At Salerno, the candidate was expected to expound freely on any lemma selected at random: *scilicet quod casu lectio vel punctus occurrebat, exponebat in aula medica* (Sudhoff, "Salerno, Montpellier und Paris im 1200," *Sudhoffs Archiv* 20: [1928] pp. 51–62).

3. This sentence contains all of the essential elements of the mediaeval *accesus ad auctores: materia, intentio, causa intentionis, utilitas, suppositio, ordo tractandi* and *titulus.*

This custom came from the Aristotelian commentators through Boethius (E. A. Quain, "The Medieval accessus ad auctores," *Traditio* 3: [1945] pp. 215–264). An identical sentence appears in Maurus' *Commentarium in Aphorismos* (*CS* 4: p. 514), where he adds:

"Olim enim tres discebantur secte quarum una discebatur empiricorum ab 'empiria' quod est 'experimentum,' vel a 'pir' quod est 'ygnis,' quia circa ignem operabantur experimenta. Alia methycorum a 'methoys' quod est 'incantatio,' quum isti soli incantationibus insistebant, vel a 'methodos' quod est extra rationem, quia omnia contra rationem faciebant. Tertia logicorum qui sunt rationabiles medici."

Frequent interchange of identical sentences and short paragraphs between our text, the *Commentarium in Aphorismos* and the *Regulae Urinarum* leaves little doubt that Maurus wrote all three, thus resolving Pazzini's uncertainty as to the authorship of the *Commentarium in Aphorismos* (Stroppiana-Minghetti, pp. 20–21). A statement referring to Methodists and Empirics can be traced back at least as far as Isidore of Seville (*Etymologiae* 4.4, see W. D. Sharpe, *Isidore of Seville: The Medical Writings* [Philadelphia, 1964], p. 55); Pazzini (Stroppiana-Minghetti, pp. 18–19) takes the statement literally that Maurus considered the Methodists and Empirics as contemporary with Hippocrates, but this view is unlikely because from Soranus and Caelius Aurelianus, Maurus must have known a good deal about the older sects, and Galen's *De Sectis Medicorum* was available in Burgundio of Pisa's Latin translation as early as 1185 (Thorndike-Kibre, col. 859). Nor is it likely that Maurus is inveighing against the Methodism and Empiricism which, through Priscian and the Aurelian-Esculapian text, had entered Gariopontus, *Passionarius* and tinctured the authentic Hippocratic teachings (*CS* 4: pp. 515–517). Puccinotti (1: p. 368) sees Maurus as a defender of Salernitan tradition against the inroads of Arabic medicine, and makes the plausible suggestion that Maurus' diatribe is actually directed against the alchemists and occultists who were active at this period, the *pseudo-medici* of our text (40.57).

4. Although Macrobius (late fourth century) still considered *medicina* as the most lowly subdivision of *physica*, by the time of Adelard (*ca.* 1110), who studied at Salerno in his youth, *medicina* and *naturalis scientia* were linked as equals "within the more comprehensive sphere of *physica*" (Lawn, p. 20). Yet at the very same period, Hugh of St. Victor (1096–1141) in his *Didascalicon* insists upon placing medicine among the mechanical or technical arts (Flint, p. 94). According to Kristeller ("*Nuove Fonti*, 11 pp. 71–72), Maurus modifies the schema of his predecessor Bartholomaeus, substituting *theoricam* for *naturalem scientiam*. *Phisica*, although still a rung lower than *theorica* in his classification, is now a distinct entity, thus anticipating the eventual divergence of physic from natural philosophy. (Phisica est scientia que agit de principio intrinseco, id est, de natura, et dividitur in tres partes, in phisicam partem, methoram (methodicam) et medicinam. B.N.Lat. 18499 lvB.) The procession from ordinary medical practice, through medicine and theory, to natural science reflects the common scholastic arrangement of all knowledge into a hierarchy presided over by theology. Guido Aretino (1170) explains that while "treatment is given us by theory, it is administered by practice," and that both these disciplines are subject to logic, of which he calls himself a supporter (Corner, "Salernitan Surgery," p. 91).

5. Maurus's threefold division (*virtus animalis* [brain], *virtus naturalis* [liver] and *virtus spiritualis* [heart]) follows the more venerable tradition of Plato and Aristotle rather than that of Galen. Indeed Siegel (pp. 186–188) doubts that the original Galenic doctrine included a *spiritus naturalis*. Each section of our text is devoted to a single virtue (see Allbutt, pp. 235, 297).

6. Galen elaborates on this theme in *Ars medica* 4 (Kühn 1.313) and *Commentary on the Prognostics* 4 (K. 18B.11, 16–17). The reference to the *Tegni* may be found in book 2, sent. 5, of *Articella nuperrime impressa* (Lyons, 1515), fol. 90.

7. That the art of prognosis was applied to the healthy as well as to the sick is evident from the Hippocratic *Art of Medicine* 13 and *Regimen* 3.69. The latter has a distinct reference to "prognosis before illness" (Jones 4.383). I believe that Maurus, whose task it was to keep the nobles of the court in good health, must have been familiar with the medical history and personal problems of his patients even before they came under his care during a specific illness.

8. Thorndike-Kibre (col. 1002) list manuscripts with this incipit as "Hippocrates Pronostica, cum commento Galieni, translated by Constantinus Africanus." Actually, as Kibre shows, the same text appears in additional manuscripts with the gloss incipit *Videtur mihi quod ex melioribus rebus* (Kibre, p. 388), listed in Thorndike-Kibre, col. 1694, as "Galen, Comm. Hippocrates, Pronostica, probably translated by Gerard of Cremona." Constantinus relates that his favorite pupil, Atto, prevailed on him to translate Galen's *Commentary on the Aphorisms*, but there is no such evidence with respect to the *Commentary on the Prognostics* (Puccinotti, 1: p. 343). Steinschneider first questions ("Constantinus," p. 407) and later denies (*Europäischen Übersetzungen*, p. 11) a Constantian translation of this work; he attributes a later anonymous translation of the *Prognostica* without a commentary to Peter the Deacon, and credits Gerard of Cremona with the version complete with translation which appears in the first printed editions. There is no evidence that Gerard's translation reached Salerno before 1200 (Lawn, p. 40). Pazzini (Stroppiana-Minghetti, pp. 11–17) argues convincingly from the many references to Galen in Maurus' *Commentary on the Aphorisms* that the latter used Galen's commentary on this work, presumably in Constantinus' translation. This does not necessarily preclude the possibility that Maurus also had access to the contemporary Greek-to-Latin translation of the *Aphorisms* by Burgundio of Pisa, even though this translation was not accompanied by Galen's commentary. Beccaria (457) lists several manuscripts of Galen's own *Prognostica* which contain the *signa mortifera*, and these may have been known to Maurus. Nevertheless, close study of our text provides no convincing evidence that Maurus was familiar with or made use of Galen's commentary on the *Prognostics* of Hippocrates in preparing his own glosses on this Hippocratic text.

9. The exact wording given by Maurus, perhaps from memory, does not appear in Lane Cooper, *A Concordance to Boethius* (Cambridge, Massachusetts, 1928). but see p. 229: *neque enim medicina aegris non semper affert salutem, sed nulla erit culpa.* Boethius completed a translation of Porphyry's *Isagoge* and the complete *Organon*

before his death, and it was probably through this source that Maurus acquired some of his first notions of Aristotelian terminology. He uses such expressions as *universalis, particularis, accidentalis, potentialis, actualis, opifex, substantia,* and *forma.* Although we have noted that Maurus and Urso were contemporaries and perhaps collaborators, it was the latter who was far more attracted to the philosophic aspects of medicine, as his surviving writings clearly demonstrate.

10. Frank recognition by a physician of the limits of his resources and termination of active measures of treatment which might add to a dying patient's discomfort has a tradition dating to antiquity; see Francis Adams, *The Seven Books of Paulus Aegineta* (London, 1844–1847) 1: pp. 501–502, and Edelstein, 1967: pp. 382–384.

11. *Cf.* Maurus's *Commentarium in Aphorismos* (*CS* 4.529): *Egritudo igitur aut habet fieri ex acumine indigestionis materie aut ex cruditate ipsius.* Fecal impaction from one cause or another seems to have contributed heavily to mortality during the Middle Ages. Dread of this complication is evident here and implied elsewhere by the countless drugs recommended for purging. The famous pills attributed to Maurus himself contain no fewer than fifty ingredients, among which the most active are aloes, senna, and the castor bean. Although recommended for such diverse conditions as paralysis, epilepsy, gout, loss of memory, and deafness, they were primarily effective as cathartics (*CS* 3: p. 51). There are two methods of purging the intestinal tract: *ab ore stomachi et a diafragmate superious, a fundo stomacho inferius* (*CS* 4: p. 521). Maurus is conservative in the use of strong purges, avoiding them on extremely hot or cold days, and during the first and third trimesters of pregnancy. He warns that in *psiticos,* the strain of vomiting may bring on pulmonary hemorrhage (*CS* 4: p. 543).

12. In *Airs, Waters, Places* 2, Hippocrates recommends that the physician acquire some knowledge of astronomy. Maurus's writings, and those of the Salernitans generally, are notably free of the influence of magic, astrology, and kindred superstititions, but like all medieval physicians, Maurus liked to demonstrate his familiarity with astronomy, mathematics, and science generally. He follows Constantinus (*Opera Conquisita* 20, 290, 356) in avoiding the new moon and dog days for phlebotomy and advocates his own theory of diurnal variations in selecting the hour for bleeding best suited for various temperaments (*CS* 4: p. 520). For each of these recommendations, however, he attempts to supply a rational explanation (Buerschaper, 1919. pp. 8–10). In discussing the ideal season of the year for purges, he relates the star *canis* to the Zodiacal sign Leo, and *anticanis* to Aquarius (*CS* 4: p. 543); see also our text 34.58 ff.

13. Our text has the classical *dignosco* (30.66, 35.22, 35.29) as well as the medieval *disgnosco* (2.53, 42.91) and *disnosco* (2.59, 36.29, 44.19). These terms are used in the sense of "to judge" or "to assess" the reaction of a specific disease on the patient, and thus differ slightly in their meaning from *pronostico* (*passim*) and *predico* (2.25, 2.27, 44.15) which refer to the terminal result or, rather, to the probable course.

14. Careful reading of the *De febribus opus sane aureum* by Constantinus (Venice, 1576) 201–206, incorrectly numbered 101–106, does not reveal this schema of the nine favorable and unfavorable signs. Maurus may have abstracted them from some other source.

15. See note 9 above.

16. Clinical jaundice can first be detected by examination of the sclerae or whites of the eyes, hence, part of the *facies*. In severe jaundice, an admixture of green with the yellow may result in a brown or black color.

17. For a discussion of the five senses as elaborated early in the Middle Ages, see Sharpe, 1964: pp. 39–40.

18. The historical development of the *signal mortifera* is traced in Ogden, 1938: pp. 107–108.

19. Although the entire face is typically flushed at the onset of bacterial pneumonia, a deeper tint of red can often be seen on the cheek of the affected side, the "malar flush." This classical sign for the localization of the disease, first described by Hippocrates, remained of diagnostic importance until well after the days of Auenbrugger and Laënnec, and has not been entirely supplanted by roentgenographic examination.

20. The text is confusing and may be defective, while the Vatican manuscript is useless as a corrective. Maurus seems to mean that there are three favorable signs: (1) the patient's features remain unchanged from what they were in health; (2) the patient's resistance matches the strength of the disease; and (3) the patient's complexion is unchanged from his normal coloring.

21. For Maurus, the body's members are either noble or ignoble, and the latter are subservient to the former, conceding heat, moisture, and nutrition to them whenever required (7.5, 17.15–17). In general, the ignoble members are exposed, the noble (liver, heart, brain) are protected, one exception to this being the spleen which is specifically characterized as ignoble (11.11).

22. Maurus uses various terms to indicate stages of inflammation: *corruptio* = suppuration, *consumptio* = atrophy, *principium mortificationis* = severe induration, *profunda mortificatio* = necrosis and *adustio* = gangrenous destruction.

23. In discussing signs to be derived from examination of the eyes, Maurus shows himself a careful observer. He postulates a close connection between the eyes and brain, and between the eyes and organs of respiration. Through the latter connection, he explains temporary protrusion of the eyeballs seen in asthmatic attacks and dyspnea; through the former, inequality in size and perhaps ptosis and irregular movements caused by insanity or paralysis. He describes exophthalmos, perhaps from thyrotoxicosis; enophthalmos, which he associates with cachexia; and corneal ulceration, a not uncommon complication of high fevers. He also describes incomplete closure of the eyelids during sleep, a common symptom of many exhausting diseases, especially in children, and associates photophobia and lachrymation with mental and nervous disorders. That these latter symptoms are frequently precursors of meningeal irritation, or "phrenitis," was well known by the ancients (Aretaeus, Adams 278; Caelius Aurelianus, Drabkin 77). Maurus accepts the heightened visual acuity attributed to the insane and advises a quiet, dark place where phrenitic patients can rest undisturbed by visitors (*CS* 4: p. 517).

24. The theory that mentally disturbed patients are insensitive to pain dates back, according to Caelius Aurelianus (Drabkin 11, 27), to Aesclepiades, and this tradition persisted until long after the time of Benjamin Rush (*ob.* 1813), thus contributing much to the cruel treatment of these unfortunates. Elsewhere (*CS* 4: pp. 550–551) Maurus elaborates:

"Estasis qui stupor appelatur et mentis insania vel alienatio cum instrumentis sensuum ad sensum paratis autem sensu privatur et ipsa deterior est mania cum ipsa sensibus omnino hominem privet."

25. Maurus uses the term *fumositas* to indicate exhalations or emanations, usually arising within the body from irritating matter or homors; thus, *fumositates* from harmful matter may irritate the eyes, extinguish the heart's heat (9.21), blunt the brain's functions, cause nausea and even lead to swelling of the abdomen. On the other hand, *fumositates* may also be released from swamps (*Commentarium super Isagoge*, BN 18499 f25). A *liquorosa fumositas* derived from food and drink moistens the brain, softens its membranes and produces sleep (*CS* 3: p. 192). At one point (23.1–18), Maurus seems to equate *fumositas* with *ventositas*. *Fumositates* had no fixed location and might be eliminated from the body through the intestines, lungs, and pores of the skin.

26. Apparently Maurus did not know the term *xerophthalmia* (Celsus 6.6.29), the Greek equivalent for *lippitudo*. See note 73 below.

27. This may refer to post-nasal drip, a frequent complication of chronic sinusitis, which leads to severe coughing when the patient awakens from sleep. Maurus uses the plural *spiritualia* when referring to the respiratory system as a functional unit, generally reserving *pulmo* for the lung as an anatomic unit.

28. The dorsal position which Maurus considers so undesirable is observed in many conditions characterized by great weakness, such as the early phase of typhoid fever. The tendency to slip forward to the foot of the bed may have been aggravated by the short medieval bed and high bolsters which kept the patient in an aggravated upright position. A rigid dorsal position with the legs drawn up often indicates marked abdominal pain and tension, usually from peritonitis. The involuntary tonic contractions which Maurus describes may be associated with cerebellar injury or disease, although the jumping spasms of hysteria and epilepsy may be confused with these. The prone position is often adopted in colic and spasm, less frequently in gastric ulcer and mediastinal disease.

29. By *frenesis*, Maurus implies a febrile delirium; by *amentia*, a mental disturbance with or without loss of consciousness. Cf. note 23.

30. That Maurus continued to use the word *nervus* loosely as an all-inclusive term for tendons and ligaments as well as nerves is apparent here and elsewhere in his writings; see, for example, the *Anatomia Mauri* (Ploss 7) and our text (43.3). This confusion persisted into the eighteenth century; cf. *Amaltheum Castello-Brunonianum* (Padua, 1746) 550: *Nervus accipitur late et stricte. Late includit, praeter nervos proprie dictos, etiam tendines et ligamenta.*

31. *Venter* here refers to the abdomen, but may refer to any bodily cavity, including the uterus, intestinal tract and the ventricles of the brain or heart.

32. Metastatic cerebral abscess from a pulmonary abscess is a complication of lobar pneumonia by no means unknown in antibiotic times.

33. Grinding of the teeth, when not deliberate, is correctly considered a symptom of disease of the central nervous system in adults, and a complication of high fevers among children.

34. Subsultus tendinum, carpholalgia, and related symptoms here described by Maurus were regarded by the ancients as serious portents of agonal decerebration; see Galen (K. 18B.73), Aretaeus (Adams 272) and Caelius Aurelianus (Drabkin 23). These signs were commonly noted in the 'typhoid status' of our grandfathers.

35. Maurus again shows excellent powers of observation and description in this section. Among the entities which may tentatively be identified are the hypercapnea associated with emphysema and other forms of cardio-pulmonary disease, the deep rapid breathing of acidosis, the hyperventilation of the tense and anxious patient and the rapid, shallow breathing of metabolic alkalosis which may follow severe vomiting.

36. The Enigmatic phrase *luna caloris* is found again in the Dresden manuscript of the *De flebotomia*, but the Brussels manuscript reads, in discussing *causon: quia est ibi actuissimus calor propter siccitatem incertam, quae est lima caloris* (Buerschaper, 1919: p. 20). Dryness is therefore a polishing or refinement of heat.

37. Maurus here and elsewhere (*CS* 4: p. 513) pays tribute to the ancients' greater medical learning and knowledge of anatomy. In his own day at Salerno, public dissection seems to have been limited to the pig and his own anatomical treatise, the so-called *Third Salernitan Demonstration*, is clearly derived from the *Pantegni* (Corner, "Anatomical Texts," pp. 29–30). This may have been a youthful effort, because our present manuscript and the *Regulae Urinarum* demonstrate advanced anatomical knowledge. Pazzini, 1944: **1**: p. 417, finds close agreement between the anatomical knowledge of the *Regulae Urinarum* and the *Anatomia Mauri*.

38. *Alienatio spiritus* probably refers to Cheyne-Stokes respiration, a form of breathing marked by respirations which gradually increase in depth to a peak and then decrease, ceasing entirely for a short interval, until the cycle resumes or death supervenes.

39. Maurus elaborates at considerable length on the prognostic value of sweat in his *Commentarium in Aphorismos* (*CS* 4: pp. 530–550). The dangerous implication of a cold sweat affecting the head and neck such as is often observed in cardiovascular collapse following myocardial infarction or acute cardiac failure is here noted.

40. For the significance of *phlegma* in Galenic physiology, see Siegel, 1968: pp. 223, 322–332. Galen describes two varieties, the sweet and sour (acid), and to these (*dulce et salsum*), Maurus adds natural phlegm or mucus and bitter phlegm (*acerbum*), the latter derived from an excess of bile. See our text, 21.13–20.

41. Hippocrates used the terms "right hypochondria" and "left hypochondria" to designate that part of the upper abdomen particularly protected by the costal cartilages. Copho and the author of the second anonymous Salernitan text on anatomy (probably Bartholomaeus) both follow this usage, as did Urso later on (Sudhoff, "Die vierte Salernitaner Anatomie," *Archiv. f. Gesch. d. Medizin* **20** [1928]: pp. 33–50). Only Maurus speaks of the two hypochondria as "concavities" divided into four quadrants, two above the diaphragm and two below. This seems to be an original concept, probably adopted in teaching for ease of diagnostic localization and demonstration. It was not accepted by later writers, and the term *hypochondrium* itself soon fell into disuse and is no longer to be found in versions of the 13th century *Anatomia Nicolai* and the *Anatomia Ricardi* as published by Corner ("Anatomical Texts," pp. 67–110).

42. The text is confusing. Maurus places the lung in the right superior hypochondrium, but the liver in the left superior hypochondrium. This must be a scribal transposition of *epar* for *cor;* see our text 4.28–29: *cor positum in sinistro latere* and 11.12: *si esset in sinistro superiori pessimum esset quia ibi est cor.* The spleen is correctly located in the lower left hypochondrium, but the situation of the liver is not here defined. In the *Anatomia Mauri* (Ploss 8), we read: *Ibidem invenitur stomachus inter splenem et epar locatus, splen in sinistra, epar in dextra suppositum stomacho.* The text is accordingly corrected despite lack of MS authority.

43. Maurus confirms the ominous significance given by Hippocrates (*Prognosis* 7) to right-sided involvement of the abdomen, often interpreted as an early reference to appendicitis.

44. *Cor . . . membrum ad vitam destinatum* suggests that Maurus embraced without reservation Galen's argument from design. The utility of each organ and part is expounded in Galen's *De usu partium*, and because this utility brought Galen to postulate the existence and operations of a Designer, his doctrine found wide acceptance by the mediaeval theologian and scientist alike. Elsewhere in our text (40.7), Maurus describes the uvula as *membrum a natura deputatum.* For a brief discussion of Galenic teleology, see Brock, 1929: pp. 28–29. See also our text 15.101–104, 24.8–11.

45. Maurus attempts to reconcile divergent positions of two authorities on the nature of abscesses derived from blood. He postulates an unnatural ichor or extravasated blood as the basis for the soft abscess of Hippocrates, although Hippocratic writings do not refer to the two varieties of blood. The "cold abscess" of Johannitius here cited has a slow development without obvious signs of inflammation, and is notoriously painless. It is usually of tuberculous origin.

46. The doctrine of "praiseworthy" or "laudable" pus which was to persist until the era of Pasteur and Lister is here expounded. Maurus obviously did not consider all varieties of pus equally salutary, yet at the very time that he wrote, the barbarous seton, previously advocated by Paul of Aegina and Rhases to induce suppuration and healing by tertiary intention was being reintroduced into Europe through the influential *Practica Chirurgiae* of Maurus's colleague, Roger of Salerno. See Mettler, 1947: p. 832, and out text 14.23 ff.

47. Maurus attempts to differentiate between several varieties of cutaneous infections: (1) the acute, superficial, sharply pointed furuncle; (2) the more deeply situated suppuration known as a carbuncle; and (3) the malignant cellulitis known as "phlegmona diffusa" which pits freely on pressure, is frequently associated with lymphangitis, metastatic abscesses and general sepsis, and often runs a fatal course.

48. Apparently twelfth-century Salerno still regarded Gariopontus's compilation as a reflection of the authentic teachings of Galen. The reference to the *Viaticum* may be found in *Viaticum Ysaac . . . quod Constantinus sibi attribuitur* in Isaac Judaeus, *Opera Omnia* (Lyons, 1515) fol. 160rB: *Ydropisis est errare virtutem in epate naturalem: virtus enim digestiva epatis.* *Cf.* Galeni Pergameni, *Opera Omnia* (Basel, 1536) 118.38: *Causa vero cuiusque hydropis est, auctore Erasistrato, inflammatio iecinoris et lienis, temporis spatium in scirrhum indurata,* and *Passionarius Galeni Guaripontus* (Lyons, 1526), fol. 43rA: *Hydrops est extensio ventris ultra modum naturale ex aquoso atque corrupto humore effecta,* continuing (fol. 43vA) that the liver is but one of a number of organs causing dropsy and (fol. 43vB) that the liver swells with dropsy. This is apparently a reference to the ascites of hepatic cirrhosis, most frequently associated with chronic alcoholism, then as now. Neither Gariopontus nor Galen defines *hydrops* exactly as does Maurus, but Constantinus (or Isaac) is quoted correctly. See our note 82 below. Siegel, 1968: pp. 334–339, discusses Galen's views on dropsy, and finds that he considered the kidneys rather than the liver to be the principal organ involved.

49. Maurus here makes a subtle distinction: although dropsy is quite clearly stated to arise from some defect of the liver's function, it is not to be considered a defect of the liver itself.

50. Maurus discusses ascites at greater length than any other single pathologic entity. Aside from including tympanites as a form of dropsy (*CS* **4**: p. 544), *Ydropem siccum id est timpanitem,* Maurus's classification is accurate. The terms *gibbum* and *syma* used respectively for the convexity and portal surface of the liver, and the terms *siphac* and *zirbac* for the peritoneum and omentum, are all derived from the Arabic. Maurus describes the omentum in some detail in his *Commentarium in Aphorismos* (*CS* **4**: p. 545), indicating correctly its attachment to the pyloric end of the stomach (*portonarius*), duodenum, spleen, kidneys and liver. Although Maurus considers liver disease the primary cause of dropsy, he appreciates that in advanced cases, the lungs, spleen, and kidneys are also involved (see our text 15.74–126). Before Harvey's proof of the circulation of the blood, Maurus could not have been aware of the role of the failing heart in the development of ascites. All things considered, portal hypertension from hepatic cirrhosis remains the commonest cause of ascites in day-to-day medical practice.

51. The hollow veins, or *venae cavae,* are so called because they are usually found empty after death. Aetius of Amida (sixth century) attributes their original description to Diogenes, see Skinner, 1949: p. 362.

52. Another description of portal hypertension.

53. *Phisis* is here used as a synonym for *natura:* the fine distinction sometimes made by such contemporary philosophical writers as Bernard Silvestre between the Greek *physis* and the Latin *natura* does not seem to exist for Maurus, who uses the terms indiscriminately. For a discussion of *physis,* see Brock, 1929: p. 3.

54. For an elaboration of Maurus's interpretation of coughing as related to dropsy, see his *Commentarium in Aphorismos* (*CS* **4**: p. 553).

55. Maurus mentions the pores several times as organs of insensible respiration whereby the body eliminate-noxious by-products. This concept began with Empedocles and the Sicilian school, and was revived by later Methodists, especially Themison. Galen uses *poros* in two ways: to describe the anatomic pores of the skin and as a synonym for *meatus* with special reference to the passage of the *sensibilis spiritus* over the *nervus opticus* (Allbutt, 1921: pp. 104, 193). Isidore of Seville includes the pores of the skin among the organs of respiration (Sharpe, 1964: p. 44). Maurus explains his own views in *Regulae Urinarum* (*CS* **3**: p. 2):

"Fluxui quod cotidie corpus humanum fluit tam per manifestos quam per occultos poros. Per manifestos utpote oculorum pictuitate, aurium superfluitate, narium muccilagine, oris sputo, minctu urine, et ventris obsequio; per occultos ut per sudorem, per pilorum emissiones, et per varias corporis respirationes."

And in his discussion of various methods of purgation (*CS* **4**: p. 521), Maurus notes: *si secundum cutem caraxationibus, sudoribus et aliis respirationibus.*

56. Maurus distinguishes between the cyanotic fingernails of cardiac disorders, such as cor pulmonale and certain congenital anomalies, and the yellowish discoloration attributable to liver failure accompanied by jaundice.

57. Antonius Musa, who flourished at Rome under Augustus, was the most famous of the emperor's physicians and a noted advocate of cold bathing. Sarton, 1927: **1**: p. 231, states that his famous work on materia medica, *De herba vettonica,* cited by Galen, is lost but that spurious versions circulated widely under his name during the Middle Ages. Beccaria, 1956: p. 440, lists no fewer than fifteen Latin and two Anglo-Saxon manuscripts of the work; Durling, 1967: p. 424, three sixteenth-century editions.

58. Complete shedding of the nails may occur after severe febrile reactions, particularly after scarlet fever.

59. The testes are often retracted in peritonitis and in strangulated herniae.

60. By the *membrum offiitiale* adjacent to the penis, Maurus may refer to the prostate gland.

61. The Salernitans, contrary to the ancients, seem to have regarded the testes as less noble than the liver, heart and brain, presumably because a eunuch, though deprived of these male organs, continues to live (Desnos 61).

62. Maurus has much to say about sleep in his *Commentarium in Aphorismos* (*CS* **4**: pp. 537–538) where he attempts to distinguish between normal refreshing sleep and other forms of loss of consciousness, such as the somnolence or lethargy seen in phrenitis and paralysis. Maurus considers sleep beneficial for the insane, but those who toss about excessively during sleep are dangerously ill.

63. Usually Maurus uses *mortificatio* to designate necrosis, a stage before *adustio,* which implies complete and permanent destruction. Here, however, *mortificatio* seems to indicate a "resemblance to death" from excessive use of opium, hence, profound coma.

64. The Aristotelian terms *congregativa* and *disgregativa* may have come to Maurus through Boethius, who used them in his commentary on the *Topica.* See Souter, 1949: pp. 72, 108.

65. The text is defective at this point, items two and three of Maurus's list having dropped out.

66. Maurus here refers to his own glosses on the *Aphorisms*, indicating that these already existed when the Commentary on the *Prognostics* was prepared. The discussion of dysentery is at *CS* 4: p. 518.

67. The incident of Galen, the enema and the heroic procedure required to relieve the impaction are found in the *Ars medica* (K. 1.391). The tarry stool and inability to retain food in this case may have been due to uremia, or more probably to an obstructive tumor of the gastrointestinal tract.

68. Worms were probably considered a favorable sign because gastrointestinal distress caused by them is of a non-malignant origin, hence rarely fatal. The theory of spontaneous generation, first seriously attacked by Spallanzani (1765), was finally put to rest through the investigations of Louis Pasteur.

69. Paranoid schizophrenic women are still frequently deluded by the idea that they harbor reptiles in their wombs.

70. The four species of worms described by Maurus probably include *Taenia solium* and *Ankylostoma duodenale*, common throughout the Mediterranean littoral; the round worm, *Ascaris lumbricoides*, common among children, and the pinworm, *Oxyuris vermicularis*, which frequently invades the pudic circle and the vagina.

71. Blackish, liquid stools, the dark red-gray of prune juice, may be due to blackwater diarrhea, a frequently fatal complication of malaria. For this and other suggestions relating to tropical medicine, gratitude is due Dr. Heracleo Alabado y Magbanua, formerly of the Philippines.

72. *Oxeum*, more commonly *oscheum* or *oschium:* Maurus combines a Greek term, ὀχεὸν, with a Latin termination and—as elsewhere— deliberately uses a Greek form rather than the commoner Latin form. Celsus states (7.18): ὀσχεὸν *Graeci, scrotum nostri vocant.* Isidore of Seville used Greek-Latin medical glosses in preparing his work, and Maurus probably had similar word lists. Confusion between Greek χ and Latin x documents poor Greek scholarship; see Sharpe, 1964: pp. 14–15.

73. This extended discussion of the urine as a diagnostic tool reflects not only the general medieval interest in uroscopy but, more particularly, Maurus's interest in this subject. His *Regulae Urinarum*, although hardly an original work, was by far his most influential (see Introduction, note 92). For a full discussion of urology and uroscopy during the Middle Ages, the best sources remain Vieillard and Desnos, cited in the bibliography.

74. Desnos, 1914: pp. 59–61, credits Maurus with the concept, later made popular by Gilles, that the urine reflects the condition of the liver. This organ, the seat of the nutritive faculty, was considered by the Salernitans as primordial, that is, as existing before the soul entered the body and thus the foundation and root of the human structure.

75. *Pir* occurs in Isidore of Seville, *Etymologiae* 10.129, 2.12.6, 15.11.4 and 16.1.9 (see Sharpe, 1964: p. 18). Sharpe considers this a variant form of πῦρ, *fire,* suggesting

that it is a good Latin word not yet incorporated into the usual glossaries.

76. The Salernitans, like the Greeks before them, distinguished carefully between the acute, mainly malarial, fevers and the protracted *ethica*, or hectic fever. Because a hectic fever accompanies typhoid fever, tuberculosis, the terminal cachexia of malignant disease and other conditions, with grave prognoses, Maurus's frank pessimism is readily understandable. Elsewhere (*CS* 3: p. 45), Maurus elaborates his views of hectic fevers, giving the following definition:

"Ethica febris est febris in principali vitio membrorum proveniens. Dicitur autem ethica ab ethis, quod est habitus; eo quod adveniens corpori in habitum convertitur."

Maurus describes three varieties of hectic fever depending on whether the fever exacerbates before or after meals or at both times. Here, he considers the second and third varieties to be fatal, although supplying a *cura*. Elsewhere in our text (42.47), Maurus refers to still another distinct variety of fever, the drawn-out *interpolata* or intermittent, characterized by long periods of remission and carrying a much more favorable prognosis.

77. This description might equally refer to diabetes mellitus or to diabetes insipidus. Both are especially apt to be fatal among children, and the latter may arise from a posterior fossa brain tumor.

78. References to a syndrome characterized by oily or fatty matter in the urine and deposits which look like spider-webs on the surface of the voided urine, accompanied by general wasting, might be related to nephrosis or to the nephrotic syndrome.

79. Maurus distinguishes between urinary deposits incident to systemic renal disease and to the fetid sediment full of epithelial cells found in cystitis and other vesical diseases, including cancer, and often associated with yellowish calculi.

80. Elsewhere (*CS* 4: p. 543), Maurus discusses ease of vomiting in relationship to bodily habitus and complexion, using the phrase *purgare superiora, id est per superiores regiones*, and again (*CS* 4: p. 550) notes that excessive vomiting with singultus may rupture the vessels of the eyes.

81. Maurus does not clearly differentiate between an inflammation of the pleura alone and involvement of the lung parenchyma proper. He correctly refers to a wet pleurisy (*empyema*), but insists that a peripneumonia ("dry pleurisy") does not directly invade the lungs, nor, following Hippocrates and Galen, does he ever use the term *pneumonia*. Perhaps the fact that he could observe the continuation of an orderly, although accelerated, process of respiration led him to this conclusion. From his remark (28.16), it seems clear that the subject was already controversial. See also his *Regulae Urinarum* (*CS* 3: p. 35): *Collectio in pleura et in pulmonis casula, et speciali vocabulo dicitur "pleuresis," alia circa pulmonem et "peripleumonia" vocatur*, and again (*CS* 3: p. 37): *Peripleumonia est apostema quod fit in pulmone scilicet in pulmonis casula et non in ipsa pulmonis substantia, ut quidam dicunt*. Siegel, 1968: pp. 326–327, considers that the Hippocratic *peripneumonia* (Coan Prognosis 394) does imply consolidation of lung tissue, but that this entity may have differed from our classical lobar pneumonia of pre-antibiotic days.

82. Earlier in his text (15.9–10), Maurus attributed the *Viaticum* to Constantinus. Does this present attribution to Isaac indicate that the plagiarism of Constantinus was already recognized in Maurus's day? We know now that the work which went under the name of *Viaticum Constantini* and which was later attributed to Isaac Judaeus in his *Opera Omnia* (Lyons, 1515) is actually a free translation of the work of Ibn-al-Jazzar, a pupil of Israëli. The reference is to book 3, chapter 12 (fol. cliiiᵛ B):

"Pleuresis non vera habet haec signa; gravitatem lateris sine tussi, nullum screatum emittit, quia morbus extra spiritus instrumentum existit; locus exterior manu tactus dolorem parit infirmo, aliquando extra apparet tumor."

83. An early reference to the body as a machine: Maurus may have had a pre-Cartesian vision of bodily function as an essentially mechanical process. LaMettrie quotes both Hippocrates and Galen to support his own doctrine.

84. As might be expected from an advocate of the theory of diurnal variation of the humors, Maurus places extraordinary importance on the precise hour as well as the day on which the earliest symptoms of a disease first make their appearance. The terms used by Maurus and the other Salernitans in describing the course of an illness are as follows: *Initium* = first symptom, before the onset of the fever—this is an important diagnostic point in determining when the crisis will arrive; *Principium* = fever begins; *Augmentum* = rise in bodily temperature and accentuation of symptoms; *Status* = height of the disease process; *Declinatio* = gradual amelioration; and *Expulsio* = complete elimination of waste products and resolution of the disease. In those illnesses which are marked by a *crisis*, this event would occur immediately after the *status*, and should be accompanied by very rapid elimination and recovery from the ailment. See our text 44.28–29.

85. Maurus mentions the soul in this text on several occasions (18.27, 19.17, 19.44 and 20.91). The soul is closely tied to the body by the humors and spirits as bonds, and is not released until these are completely destroyed. The soul performs certain functions in the interior of the body during the day, but leaves for the exterior at night. Maurus thus seems familiar with the ancient belief, restated by Plato, that in respect to this tendency, sleep has an affinity with death.

86. Malformation of the fingernails of this kind occurs in cardiopulmonary osteoarthropathy. Multiple septic emboli could explain the small, recurrent abscesses noted in the feet.

87. Vesico-pustular eruptions may appear in apparently normal skin from secondary infection when the antecedent systemic disease is of sufficient intensity to seriously weaken the patient's general bodily defenses.

88. This fanciful reference to the stomach as *paterfamilias* or chief provider is echoed by Alexander Neckham, thus providing another link with Gilles and Salerno. Thomas Wright, ed. *Alexandri Neckam De Naturis Rerum* (London, 1863), p. 274.

89. Suppurative parotitis is occasionally observed during the course of typhoid fever and other infectious diseases associated with dehydration, including pneumonia. It may have been a more frequent complication in the warm, dry climates of southern Italy and Greece.

90. This may refer to bacterial meningitis following an extremely painful suppurative otitis media or sinusitis.

91. "Wet," or infectious, gangrene with loss of toes or of an entire foot was not uncommon following typhoid or scarlet fever during pre-antibiotic days.

92. This firm substance may be an organized blood clot. Pressure on the urinary bladder may come from a rectal or prostatic tumor which invades the pelvis.

93. Maurus here seems to refer to the symptoms of malignant tumors of the rectum and sigmoid colon, and perhaps to the "shelf metastasis" or "drop metastasis" from a tumor higher in the abdominal cavity which forms a hard ridge feeling much like the edge of a shelf when examined by a finger passed into the anus.

94. In the Greek system of counting days, the initial day is included in the total; thus, the day after tomorrow becomes the third day. This custom is reflected in the terms "tertian" and "quartan," and is accepted by Maurus without comment. In Italian, "a week from today" remains *oggi otto*.

95. Hippocrates, *Prognostics* 20, relating to the critical day in acute diseases has been the subject of much controversy and confusion. By a bit of scholastic reasoning, Maurus attempts to smooth away these difficulties. While demonstrating his knowledge of astronomy and mathematics, he also impresses his students with his familiarity with the writings of the ancients. Because according to Maurus, we may reckon by an incomplete or imperfect number as well as by one which is complete or perfect, the crisis may come at almost any time, and still conform to the prediction. One may perhaps comment that Maurus was far from the last medical lecturer to display irrelevant erudition to explain away inconsistent data.

96. Hippocrates, *Aphorisms* 2.23: Acute diseases come to a crisis in fourteen days.

97. The varieties of pain described by Maurus, and their humoral derivation (*CS* 4: pp. 539–540) are:

Infixivus	Sanguis	*Aggrativus*	Melancolia
Pungitivus	Colera	*Deambulativus*	Ventositas
Extensivus	Flegma	*Congelativus*	Frigiditas

98. That the brain and not the heart is the controlling center of human faculties was widely appreciated by mediaeval scholars, from the Church fathers downward.

99. Maurus may refer to the staphylococcal parotitis and otitis media which, before the antibiotic era, were often complications of erysipelas in aged patients. Youths are here called "hot and dry" in contrast to Chap. 33 where Maurus speaks twice of their "great humidity."

100. Although the meaning is not altogether clear, this "incision to prevent choking" probably does not refer to tracheostomy. It may refer to an incision through the abscess itself, with evacuation of its contents. Nevertheless, the operation of opening the trachea was described as having been performed by Paul of Aegina and by Antyllus (Skinner, 1949: p. 349). The use of opium as an analgesic is to be noted. The Arabic preference for the cautery over the knife is evident, but ancient cauteries generally were shaped like a coin and thus had a cutting edge when heated.

101. Not a true tuberculosis, but a chronic pulmonary abscess. The *Viaticum* (book 3, ch. 7, folio 52vB) describes phthisis and peripneumonia together, indicating that the author had not clearly distinguished between the two processes, although the treatment then was about the same.

102. Maurus seems acutely aware of the connection between an infection of some duration and metastatic involvement of the joints. In younger people, this might manifest itself as an acute articular rheumatism, with subsidence of gross symptoms upon resolution of the abscess, the knees and ankles being the joints most frequently affected. In older people, a chronic rheumatoid arthritis may persist with frequent exacerbations of pain and fever, and monoarticular arthritides still follow gonorrheal urethritis.

103. Evidently there is some confusion between the original Hippocratic text and that used by Maurus. Referring to abscesses of the joints, the Jones translation of the *Prognosis* (2: pp. 49–50) reads: "Such abscessions come more often, and earlier when patients are under thirty" and "in older patients it (abscession) is less likely." Maurus seems to take the opposite view, that they are less apt to occur below the age of forty-five than above. Because Maurus claims to be quoting directly from Hippocrates, a scribal error or mistranslation is more likely than any genuine difference of opinion.

104. Elsewhere (*CS* 4: pp. 527–528), Maurus elaborates a theory of paroxysm in malarial fevers in which the season of the year, the hour of the day and the nature of the harmful matter involved (phlegm, bile, etc.) contribute to determine the *status* (see note 84 above) of the disease, that is, its progress to full development. Here, his description of erratic attacks fits best with that of a mixed malarial infection, that is, of an infection by two or more distinct strains of parasites, such as both tertian and quartan or estivo-autumnal malaria.

105. Maurus notes that malarial fevers tend to abate during cold weather.

106. Hippocrates, *Aphorisms* 4.59.

107. A reference to the cells or ventricles of the brain. Gilles de Corbeil speaks of an anterior cell where sanguine humors predominate, and of a posterior cell where the phlegmatic humors predominate (Vieillard, 1903: p. 289).

108. This probably describes the febrile convulsions of infancy and early childhood, although cholera infantum and marasmus may be intended. Maurus mentions that these convulsions cease at age seven: in fact, they typically do so, apparently with maturation of the thermoregulatory centers of the hypothalamus cerebri.

109. Unlike Galen, who is said to have been taught by his father to despise honor and glory, Maurus emphasizes these very rewards as an inducement to the study of medicine. From Gilles de Corbeil, we have already learned that Maurus restricted his practice to the nobles of the court and to such others as could afford handsome fees for his advice and medications.

110. It has often been remarked that Greek medicine seems to concern itself almost exclusively with those suffering from acute illness. Maurus here emphasizes that the chronic invalid must not be neglected. Although the physician should certainly familiarize himself with the prevalent diseases and seasonal variations, he must be prepared for the unusual case which may crop up unexpectedly at the "wrong" time of the year. These are the common-sense reflections of a very experienced practitioner.

111. In this final passage, Maurus again pays respect to Hippocrates as a prophetic spirit and inveighs against the quacks who follow false theories. He places Hippocrates in Ethiopia (Africa), the north (Italy) and the west (Spain) instead of in Libya, Delos, and Scythia, as found in the text of the *Aphorisms*.

BIBLIOGRAPHY

ACKERMANN, J. C. G. ed. 1970. *Regimen Sanitatis Salerni sive Scholae Salernitanae de conservanda bona valetudine praecepta* (Stendal).

ALLBUTT, T. C. 1921. *Greek Medicine in Rome* (London).

Amaltheum Castello-Brunonianum sive Lexicon Medicum. 1746. Bartholomeus Castello and Jacob Pancratus Bruno eds. (Padua).

ANSCHUTZ, WILLY. 1919. *Zwei Fieberschriften des Breslauer Codex...* (Leipzig).

ARETAEUS THE CAPPADOCIAN. 1856. *The Extant Works*, ed. and tr., Francis Adams (London).

ARTELT, WALTER. 1956. "Die Salernoforschung im 17, 18 und 19 Jahrhundert." *Sudhoffs Archiv f. Gesch. d. Medizin* **40**: pp. 211–230.

Articella nuperrime impressa cum quamplurimis tractatibus pristine impressioni superadditis... 1515 (Lyons).

AUGELLUZZI, GIUSEPPE. 1853. *Intorno ad alcuni maestri della scuola Salernitana del XII e XIII Secolo* (Naples).

BARBIERI, LUIGI, ed. 1867. *Lorenzo Rusio: La Mascalcia* (2 v., Bologna).

BARIÉTY, MAURICE, and CHARLES COURY. 1963. *Histoire de la Médicine* (Paris).

BAYON, P. 1953. "The Masters of Salerno and the Origins of the Professional Medical Practice." *Science, Medicine and History...* v.1, pp. 203–219. *Essay in Honor of Charles Singer* (London).

BECCARIA, AUGUSTO. 1956. *I Codici di Medicina del Periodo Presalernitano* (secoli ix, x e xi) (Rome).

—— 1959. "Sulle Tracce di un Antico Canone Latino di Ippocrate e di Galeno." *Italia Medioevale e Umanistica* **2**: pp. 1–56.

BIRKENMAJER, A. 1930. "Le Rôle joué par les médecins et les naturalistes dans la réception d'Aristote au XII° et XIII° siècles." *La Pologne au VI° Congrès International des Sciences Historiques*, Oslo, 1928 (Warsaw), pp. 1–15.

BLOEDNER, KARL. 1925. *Petronus, Petronius, Petroncellus, ein Salernitanischer Arzt der Mitte des 12.Jahr* (Leipzig).

Boethius: The Theological Tractates, tr. H. F. Stewart and E. K. Rand (Cambridge, Massachusetts).

BROCK, A. J. 1929. *Greek Medicine* (London).

BUERSCHAPER, RUDOLF. 1919. *Ein bisher unbekannter Aderlasstraktat des Salernitaner Arztes Maurus: "De Flebotomia"* (Borna-Leipzig).

BULLOUGH, V. L. 1966. *The Development of Medicine as a Profession: The Contribution of the Medieval University to Modern Medicine* (Basel).

CAELIUS AURELIANUS. 1950. *On Acute Diseases and On Chronic Diseases*, ed. and tr. I. E. Drabkin (Chicago).

CALVANICO, RAFFAELE, ed. 1962. *Fonti per la Storia della Medicina e della Chirurgia per il Regno di Napoli nel Periodo Angioino* (Naples).

CAPPARONI, PIETRO. 1923. "*Magistri Salernitani nondum cogniti.*" (London).

CHOLMELEY, H. P. 1912. *John of Gaddesden and the Rosa Medicinae* (Oxford).

CHOULANT, LUDWIG, ed. 1826. *Aegidii Corboliensis Carmina Medica* (Leipzig).

CONSTANTINUS AFRICANUS. 1576. In: *De febribus opus sane aureum* (Venice).

—— 1536. *Opera, Conquisita* (Basel).

CORNER, G. W. 1927. *Anatomical Texts of the Earlier Middle Ages* (Washington).

—— 1931. "The Rise of Medicine at Salerno in the Twelfth Century." *Annals Med. Hist.*, N. S. **3**: pp. 1–16.

—— 1937. "Salernitan Surgery in the Twelfth Century." *Brit. Jour. Surg.* **25**: pp. 84–99.

COTURRI, ENRICO. 1966. "La Biblioteca di un Chirurgo Toscano nel Trecento." *Pag. Stor. Med.* **10**: no. 1 pp. 77–84.

CREUTZ, RUDOLF. 1929. "Der Arzt Constantinus Africanus von Monte Cassino," *Stud. Mitt. Gesch. Bened. Ordens* **47**: pp. 1–44.

—— 1934. "Urso der Letzte des Hochsalerno, Arzt, Philosoph, Theologe." *Abhandlungen zur Gesch. der Medizin und Naturwissenschaften* **5** (Berlin).

—— 1938. "Die Medizin im Speculum Maius des Vincentius von Beauvais." *Sudhoffs Archiv f. Gesch. d. Medizin* **31**: pp. 297–313.

CREUTZ, RUDOLF, and JOHANNES STEUDEL. [1948]. *Einführung in die Geschichte der Medizin, Einzeldarstellungen* (Iserlohn).

DAREMBERG, CHARLES. 1865. *La Médecine: Histoire et Doctrines* (Paris).

—— 1870. *Histoire des Sciences Médicales* (2 v., Paris).

DERENZI, SALVATORE. 1852–1859. *Collectio Salernitana* (5 v., Naples).

—— 1857. *Storia Documentata della Scuola Medica di Salerno* (2nd ed., Naples).

DELISLE, LÉOPOLD. 1868. *Le Cabinet des Manuscrits de la Bibliothèque Impériale* (Paris) **1**: p. 306.

DESNOS, E. 1914. *Histoire de l'Urologie* (Paris).

DICKSON, CHARLES. 1934. "Le Cardinal Robert de Courson: Sa Vie." *Archives d'Histoire doctrinale et littéraire du Moyen Age* **9**: pp 53–142.

DIEPGEN, PAUL. 1911. *Gualteri Agilonis Summa Medicinalis* (Leipzig).

DINAUX, ARTHUR. 1864. *Catalogue de la Collection du Feu M. Arthur Dinaux* (Paris).

DORVEAUX, PAUL. 1906. *L'Antidotaire Nicolai* (Paris).

—— 1913. *Le Livre des Simples Medecines* (Paris).

DUBREUIL-CHAMBARDEL, LOUIS. 1914. *Les Médecins dans l'ouest de la France au XI° et XII° Siècles* (Paris). *In: Public. de la soc. française d'histoire de la med.*, No. 2, 1914, pp.1–292.

DUBREUIL-CHAMBARDEL, L., and E. WICKERSHEIMER. 1921. *Liber Memorialis Premier Congrès de l'Art de Guérir* (Antwerp).

DURLING, R. J., ed. 1967. *Catalogue of Sixteenth Century Printed Books in the National Library of Medicine* (Bethesda, Maryland).

EDELSTEIN, LUDWIG. 1967. *Ancient Medicine: Selected Papers*, ed. Owsei and C. Lillian Temkin (Baltimore).

FLINT, ROBERT. 1904. *Philosophy as Scientia Scientiarum and a History of the Classification of the Sciences* (Edinburgh).

FONAHN, ADOLF. 1922. *Arabic and Latin Anatomical Terminology Chiefly from the Middle Ages* (Kristiana).

FORT, G. F. 1883. *Medical Economy during the Middle Ages* (New York).

FRIEDENWALD, HARRY. 1944–1946. *The Jews and Medicine* (3 v., Baltimore).

FULGINEO, GENTILIS de. 1514. *Super Prima seu Quarti Canonis Avicennae* (Venice).

GALEN. 1821–1833. *Opera*, ed. K. G. Kühn (20 v., Leipzig).

GARIOPONTUS. 1526. *Passionarius Galeni* (Lyons).

GARRISON, F. H., ed. 1926. *Essays in the History of Medicine* (New York).

GARUFI, C. A. 1922. *Necrologio del Liber Confratrum di S. Matteo di Salerno* (Rome).

GIACOSA, PIERO. 1901. *Magistri Salernitani nondum editi* (1 v. and atlas, Turin).

GRATTAN, J. H. G., and SINGER CHARLES. 1952. *Anglo-Saxon Magic and Medicine* (Oxford).

HAESER, HEINRICH. 1875. *Lehrbuch der Geschichte der Medizin* (3rd ed., 3 v., Jena).

HANDERSON, HENRY E. 1918. *Gilbertus Anglicus Medicine of the Thirteenth Century* (Cleveland).

HARTMANN, GEORGE FRIEDRICH F. 1919. *Die Literatur von Früh- und Hoch-Salerno* (Borna-Leipzig).

HASKINS, C. H. 1924. *Studies in the History of Mediaeval Science* (Cambridge, Massachusetts).

—— 1927. *The Renaissance of the Twelfth Century* (Cambridge, Massachusetts)

HENSCHEL, A. W. E. Th. 1853. "Il Manuscritto Salernitano." In: *Collectio Salernitano* (Naples) 2: pp. 1–71.

HIPPOCRATES. 1849. *The Genuine Works*, tr. Francis Adams (2 v., London).

Hippocrates, with an English Translation. 1923–31. Ed. W. H. S. Jones (4 v., London).

ISAAC JUDAEUS. 1515. *Omnia Opera* (Lyons).

KADNER, ALBERT. 1919. *Ein liber de urinis des Breslauer Codex Salernitanus.* (Hamburg).

KIBRE, PEARL. 1945. "Hippocratic Writings in the Middle Ages." *Bull. Hist. Med.* 18: pp. 371–412.

KLEBS, A. C. 1963. *Incunabula Scientifica et Medica* (Hildesheim).

KRISTELLER, P. O. 1945. "The School of Salerno." *Bull. Hist. Med.* 17: pp. 138–194.

—— 1955–56. "La Scuola di Salerno," Antonio Cassese, tr. *Rassegna Storica Italiana*, Anno XVI–XVII (1955–1956): pp. 3–68.

—— 1956. *Studies in Renaissance Thought and Letters* (Rome).

—— 1958. "Nuove Fonti per la Medicina Salernitana del Secolo XII." *Rassegna Storica Salernitana*, Anno XVIII (1958): pp. 61–75.

—— 1959. "Beiträge der Schule von Salerno zur Entwicklung der Scholastischen Wissenschaft im 12. Jahrhundert." *Artes Liberales:* hrsg. J. Koch [*Studien und Texte zur Geistgeschichte der Mittelalters*] 5: pp. 84–90.

KÜHLEWEIN, HUGO. 1884. "Beiträge zur Geschichte und Beurteilung der Hippokratischen Schriften. I. Zu Hippokrates' Prognosticon." *Philologus* 42: pp. 121–127.

—— 1890. "Die handschriftliche Grundlage des hippokratischen Prognostikon und eine lateinische Übersetzung desselben." *Hermes* 25: pp. 113–140.

LAWN, BRIAN. 1963. *The Salernitan Questions* (Oxford).

LUCHAIRE, ACHILLE. 1912. *Social France at the Time of Philip Augustus*, tr. E. B. Krehbiel (London).

MACKINNEY, L. C. 1937. *Early Medieval Medicine* (Baltimore).

METTLER, CECILIA C. 1947. *History of Medicine* (Philadelphia).

MEYER-STEINEG, TH., and KARL SUDHOFF. 1950. *Geschichte der Medizin im Überblick* (4th ed. rev. Bruno von Hagen, Jena).

MINIO-PALUELLO, L. 1954. "The Ars Disserendi of Adam of Balsham 'Parvipontanus.'" *Mediaeval and Renaissance Studies (Warburg Institute)* 3: pp. 116–169.

MOULIN DE, D. 1964. *De heelkunde in de vroege middeleeuwen* (Leiden).

OGDEN, MARGARET SINCLAIR, ed. 1938. *The 'Liber de Diversis Medicinis'* (London).

ONGARO, GIUSEPPE. 1968. "Gli Antidotari Salernitani," *Salerno* 2: pp. 34–38.

PAULUS AEGINETA. 1844–1847. *The Seven Books*, tr. Francis Adams (3 v., London).

PAYNE, J. F. 1904. *English Medicine in the Anglo-Saxon Times* (Oxford).

PAZZINI, ADALBERTO. 1944. *Storia della Medicina* (2 v., Milan).

—— 1962. *Storia della Medicina: Corso di Lezioni dell' anno academico 1961–1962* (Rome).

—— 1963. "Il Pensiero medico Italiano nelle Scuole di Salerno e di Bologna." *Pag. Stor. Med.* 7: pp. 14–23.

PLOSS, W. L. H. 1921. *Anatomia Mauri* (Leipzig).

PRECOPE, JOHN. 1932. *Hippocrates on Diet and Hygiene* (London).

PUCCINOTTI, FRANCESCO. 1860–1863. *Storia della Medicina* (2 v., Naples).

PUSCHMANN, THEODOR. 1902. *Handbuch der Geschichte der Medizin*, ed. Max Neuburger and Julius Pagel (3 v., Jena).

—— 1891. *A History of Medical Education* (London).

QUAIN, E. A. 1945. "The Medieval Accessus ad Auctores," *Traditio* 3: pp. 215–264.

RASHDALL, HASTINGS. 1936. *The Universities of Europe in the Middle Ages*, ed. F. M. Powicke and A. B. Emden (3 v., Oxford).

RIESMANN, DAVID. 1935. *The Story of Medicine in the Middle Ages* (New York).

SANDERUS, ANTONIUS. 1641–1644. *Bibliotheca Belgica Manuscripta* (Insulis).

SARTON, GEORGE. 1927–1947. *An Introduction to the History of Science* (3 v., Baltimore).

SCALINCI, NOE. 1941. "La Oculistica dei Maestri Salernitani." *Scritti in Onore del Prof. Capparoni in Occasione del 50° Anno di Laurea* (Turin), pp. [134]–151.

SCHIPPERGES, HEINRICH. 1955. "Die frühen Übersetzer der arabischen medizin in chronologischer Sicht." *Sudhoffs Archiv f. Gesch. d. Medizin* 39: pp. 53–93.

—— 1961. "Ideologie und Historiographie des Arabismus." *Sudhoffs Archiv f. Gesch. d. Medizin* 45: Beiheft 1, pp. 1–76.

—— 1964. "Die Assimilation der arabischen Medizin durch das lateinische Mittelalter." *Sudhoffs Archiv f. Gesch. d. Medizin*, 48: Beiheft 3.

SEIDLER, EDUARD. 1967. "Die Heilkunde des Ausgehenden Mittelalters in Paris." *Sudhoffs Archiv f. Gesch. d. Medizin*, 51: Beiheft 8.

SHARPE, W. D. 1962. "Lung Disease and the Greco-Roman Physician." *Amer. Rev. Resp. Dis.* 86: pp. 178–192.

—— 1964. Isidore of Seville: The Medical Writings." *Trans. Amer. Philos. Soc.* 54, 2.

SIEGEL, R. E. 1968. *Galen's System of Physiology and Medicine* (Basel).

SIGERIST, H. E. 1951–1961. *A History of Medicine* (2 v., New York).

—— 1930. "Fragment einer unbekannten lateinischen Uebersetzung des Hippokratischen Prognostikon." *Sudhoffs Archiv f. Gesch. d. Medizin* 23: pp. 87–90.

—— 1958. "The Latin Medical Literature of the early Middle Ages." *Jour. Hist. Med.* 13: pp. 127–146.

SINGER, CHARLES. 1917. "A review of the medical literature of the Dark Ages." *Proc. Roy. Soc. Med., Sect. Hist. Med.* 10: pp. 107–160.

SINGER, CHARLES, and DOROTHEA. 1924. The Origin of the Medical School of Salerno, The First University. . . In: *Essays-on the History of Medicine presented to Karl Sudhoff* (Zurich). pp. 121–138.

SINNO, ANDREA. 1950. *Vicende della Scuola e dell' Almo Collegio Salernitano Maestri Finora Ignorati* (Salerno).

SKARD, E. 1940. "Nemesios," In: Pauly-Wissowa, *Real-Encyclopaedie der Classischen Altertumswissenschaft*, Supp. 7 (Stuttgart).

SKINNER, H. A. 1949. *The Origin of Medical Terms* (Baltimore).

SOUTER, ALEXANDER. 1949. *A Glossary of Later Latin* (Oxford).

STEINSCHNEIDER, MORITZ. 1866. "Constantinus Africanus und Seine Arabischen Quellen." *Virchows Archiv* 37: pp. 351–410.

—— 1868. "Maurus." *Virchows Archiv* 40: pp. 91–94.

—— 1893. *Die hebräischen Übersetzungen des Mittelalters und die Juden als Dolmetscher* (2 v., Berlin).

—— 1956. *Die Europäischen Übersetzungen aus dem Arabischen bis Mitte des 17 Jahrhunderts* (Graz).

STROPPIANA, LUIGI, and RENATO MINGHETTI. trs. 1959. *Commentario algi Aforismi di Ippocrate*, introd. Adalberto Pazzini (Rome).

SUDHOFF, KARL. 1929. "Codex Fritz Paneth." *Arch. f. Gesch. der Mathematik Naturwissenschaften und der Technik* 12: pp. 2–31.

—— 1916. "Die pseudohippokratische Krankheits Prognostik nach dem Auftreten von Hautauschlägen 'Secreta Hippocratis' oder 'Capsula Eburnea' bennant." *Archiv f. Gesch. d. Medizin* 9: pp. 79–116.

—— 1928. "Die vierte Salernitaner Anatomie." *Archiv f. Gesch. d. Medizin* 20: pp. 33–50.

—— 1928. "Salerno, Montpellier und Paris um 1200." *Archiv f. Gesch. d. Medizin* 20: pp. 51–62.

—— 1929. "Salerno: ein mittelalterliche Heil- und Lehrstelle am Tyrrhenischen Meere." *Sudhoffs Archiv f. Gesch. d. Medizin* 21: pp. 43–62. [For a shorter version in English, see Garrison, F. H., ed., *Essays in the History of Medicine* (New York, 1926), pp. 229–247.]

—— 1932. "Constantin der erste Vermittler muslimischer Wissenschaft," *Archeion* 14: pp. 359–369.

TALBOT, C. H. 1967. *Medicine in Medieval England* (London).

TEMKIN, OWSEI. 1928. "Der Systematische Zusammenhang im Corpus Hippocraticum." *Kyklos* 1: pp. 9–43.

THORNDIKE, LYNN. 1923–1958. *A History of Magic and Experimental Science* (8 v., London-New York).

THORNDIKE, LYNN, and F. S. BENJAMIN, Jr., eds. 1946. *The Herbal of Rufinus* (Chicago).

THORNDIKE, LYNN, and PEARL KIBRE. 1963. *A Catalogue of Incipits of Mediaeval Scientific Writings in Latin* (revised and augmented ed., Cambridge, Massachusetts).

TRIBALET, JACQUES. 1936. *Histoire Médicale de Chartres jusqu' au XII° Siècle* (Paris).

VIEILLARD, C. 1903. *L'Urologie et les Médecins urologues dans la Médecine ancienne: Gilles de Corbeil—Sa vie, ses Oeuvres, son Poème des Urines* (Paris).

—— 1908. *Gilles de Corbeil* (Paris).

WICKERSHEIMER, ERNEST. 1936. *Dictionnaire Biographique des Médecins en France au Moyen Age* (2 v., Paris).

INDICES

(Primus numerus capitulum, secundus paginam denotat)

Spiritus visibilis 3:25 *passim*; 8:27; 19:35 42:51

Spiritus vitalis et naturalis 18:10

Sputum 10:28; 28:41 *passim*; 29:42 *passim*; 30:33–34 *passim*; 32:45; 40:49; 44:53

Squinancia 39:48–49

Status 42:51; 44:53

Stercus 20:35–36 *passim*; 29:42; 30:45; 33:46; (spumosum) 22:37; 30:45

Sternutatio 29:42

Stomachus 4:26; 6:27; 10:28; 15:32 *passim*; 16:33; 20:35–36 *passim*; 24:38; 27:40; 28:41–42 *passim*; (os stomachi) 15:31–32; 29:43; 30:44; 42:51

Stridor dentium 6:20–21 *passim*

Strophus 16:33

Subtilia 3:25; 16:34; (aërea) 24:38; (ignea) 24:38

Subductio (superfluitas primae digestionis) 20:35–36 *passim*; 23:37

Succensio 4:26 *passim*; 16:34; 17:34; 29:43; 35:47; 39:49

Sudes (sudem) 9:27

Sudor 10:28 *passim*; 33:44

Suffocatio 3:25; 4:26; 5:26; 10:28; 29:42; 39:48–49 *passim*; 40:49

Superflua 15:32 *passim*; 16:34; 20:36; 24:38; (aggregata et non depurata) 26:40; 29:42

Superfluitates 10:28; 16:33; 20:35; 23:37 *passim*; 24:37–38; 29:(tertie digestionis) 25:39; 40:49–50; 42:50; 43:52

Syma epatis 14:31–33 *passim*; 16:33

Synocha 42:51

Tempora (timpora) 3:24

Tensio 42:51

Terrestria 16:34; 24:37

Testes 18:34

Tetanus 42:129

Theorica 1:22

Torcularis 16:34

Trachea (tracea arteria) 16:33; 30:44; 39:48–49 *passim*

Tumor 11:29; 15:31 *passim*; 16:33; 39:49

Tussis (tussicula) 16:33; 28:41; 30:44 *passim*

Tympanites (timpanites) 15:31–33 *passim*

Uber mamillarum 40:49

Umbilicus 12:30

Ungues 16, 17:33–34 *passim*

Universalia et particularia 1:22

Urina 10:28; 24, 25, 26:37–40 *passim*; 33:46

Uva 40:49–50

Vena(e) 18:34; 31:45

Vena(e) capillares 15:32

Vena concava 15:32

Vena(e) inferiorae 42:51

Vena quilis 28:25; (tertius ramus) 16:33; 23:37

Vena(e) saphenae 16:33

Venter 4:26; 5:12; 6:27; 12:30; 15:31; 16:33; 21:36; 22:37; 23:37; 29:42; 43:52

Ventositas 15:31–33 *passim*; 16:33 *passim*; 23:37 *passim*; 24:38; 26:39; 30:44; 42:51

Ventricula cerebri 19:35

Vesica 25:39; 26:40 *passim*; 33:45–46 *passim*

Viae urinales 10:29; 44:53

Vigilia 3:24; 4:26; 19:35; 43:52

Virga 16:33; 18:34 *passim*; vena per virgam 16:33

Virtus 4:26; 5:4; 15:31–33

Virtus animalis 1:22; 3:23; 19:35 *passim*

Virtus appetitiva 20:35

Virtus attractiva 10:29; 15:32; 40:50

Virtus digestiva 3:23; 15:31; 20:35; 28:41

Virtus dissecatoria 33:46; (et dissolutoria) 33:46

Virtus expulsiva 10:28; 15:31–32 *passim*; 16:33; 20:35; 28:41; 29:42–43

Virtus immutativa (secunde digestionis) 24:38

Virtus naturalis 1:22; 1:28; 15:31; 19:35; 24:38

Virtus nutriens 2:24

Virtus regitiva 3:25; 4:26; 16:95

Virtus retentiva 29:42

Virtus spiritualis 1:22; 34:46

Vis naturae 7:27; 10:28; 20:35; 27:40; 28:41

Vis symptomatis (sinthomatis) 7:27; 10:28; 20:35; 27:40; 28:41; 30:45; 39:49

Visus congregativa, disgregativa 3:25

Vomitus 20:35; 27:40–41 *passim*; 32:51

Zirbum 15:32

MEMOIRS

OF THE

AMERICAN PHILOSOPHICAL SOCIETY

TRANSACTIONS

OF THE

AMERICAN PHILOSOPHICAL SOCIETY

———————

Cosimo Brunetti: Three Relations of the West Indies in 1659–1660. SUSAN HELLER ANDERSON.
Vol. 59, pt. 6, 49 pp., 2 figs., 1969. $2.00.

Ideas of Religious Toleration at the Time of Joseph II: A Study of the Enlightenment among Catholics in Austria. CHARLES H. O'BRIEN.
Vol. 59, pt. 7, 80 pp., 1969. $2.50.

The Paleolithic Cultures of Singhbhum. ASOK K. GHOSH.
Vol. 60, pt. 1, 68 pp., 4 figs., 42 pls., 8 maps, 1970. $2.50.

The Irish Cattle Bills: A Study in Restoration Politics. CAROLYN A. EDIE.
Vol. 60, pt. 2, 66 pp., 1970. $2.50.

Philosophical Lectures by Samuel Williams, LL.D., on the Constitution, Duty, and Religion of Man. Edited by MERLE CURTI and WILLIAM TILLMAN.
Vol. 60, pt. 3, 130 pp., 1970. $4.00.

Ianula: An Account of the History and Development of the Lago di Monterosi, Latium, Italy. G. EVELYN HUTCHINSON et al.
Vol. 60, pt. 4, 175 pp., 196 figs., 1970. $7.00.

The Training of an Elite Group: English Bishops in the Fifteenth Century. JOEL THOMAS ROSENTHAL.
Vol. 60, pt. 5, 54 pp., 1970. $2.50.

Maistre Nicole Oresme: Le Livre de Politiques d'Aristote. ALBERT D. MENUT.
Vol. 60, pt. 6, 392 pp., 2 figs., 1970. $10.00.

The Carnivora of the Hagerman Local Fauna (Late Pliocene) of Southwestern Idaho. PHILIP R. BJORK.
Vol. 60, pt. 7, 54 pp., 26 figs., 2 maps, 1 chart, 1970. $2.75.

Flavius Merobaudes: A Translation and Historical Commentary. FRANK M. CLOVER.
Vol. 61, pt. 1, 78 pp., 1971. $3.00.

A Political Correspondence of the Gladstone Era: The Letters of Lady Sophia Palmer and Sir Arthur Gordon, 1884–1889. J. K. CHAPMAN.
Vol. 61, pt. 2, 52 pp., 1971. $2.00.

Practical Observations on Dropsy of the Chest (Breslau, 1706). Translated and edited by SAUL JARCHO.
Vol. 61, pt. 3, 46 pp., 1971. $2.00.

Certificates of Transmission on a Manuscript of the Maqāmāt of Harīrī (Ms: Cairo, Adab, 105). PIERRE A. MacKAY.
Vol. 61, pt. 4, 81 pp., 32 figs., 1971. $4.00.

New South Wales Immigration Policy, 1856-1900. ALBERT A. HAYDEN.
Vol. 61, pt. 5, 60 pp., 1971. $2.25.

Monastic Reform in Lorraine and the Architecture of the Outer Crypt, 950-1100. WARREN SANDERSON.
Vol. 61, pt. 6, 36 pp., 23 figs., 1971. $2.00.

Lewis Evans and His Maps. WALTER KLINEFELTER.
Vol. 61, pt. 7, 65 pp., 1 map, 1971. $2.50.

The Diplomacy of the Mexican Empire, 1863–1867. ARNOLD BLUMBERG.
Vol. 61, pt. 8, 152 pp., 15 figs., 1971. $5.00.

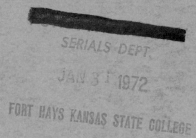
TRANSACTIONS

OF THE

AMERICAN PHILOSOPHICAL SOCIETY

HELD AT PHILADELPHIA

FOR PROMOTING USEFUL KNOWLEDGE

NEW SERIES—VOLUME 62, PART 1

1972

MAURUS OF SALERNO

Twelfth-century "Optimus Physicus"

With his Commentary on the Prognostics of Hippocrates

Now first transcribed from manuscript and
translated into English by

MORRIS HAROLD SAFFRON, M.D.

Lecturer in Medical History, Rutgers Medical School

THE AMERICAN PHILOSOPHICAL SOCIETY

INDEPENDENCE SQUARE

PHILADELPHIA

January, 1972

PUBLICATIONS

OF

The American Philosophical Society

The publications of the American Philosophical Society consist of PROCEEDINGS, TRANSACTIONS, MEMOIRS, and YEAR BOOK.

THE PROCEEDINGS contains papers which have been read before the Society in addition to other papers which have been accepted for publication by the Committee on Publications. In accordance with the present policy one volume is issued each year, consisting of six bimonthly numbers, and the price is $5.00 net per volume.

THE TRANSACTIONS, the oldest scholarly journal in America, was started in 1769 and is quarto size. In accordance with the present policy each annual volume is a collection of monographs, each issued as a part. The current annual subscription price is $15.00 net per volume. Individual copies of the TRANSACTIONS are offered for sale. This issue is priced at $4.00.

Each volume of the MEMOIRS is published as a book. The titles cover the various fields of learning; most of the recent volumes have been historical. The price of each volume is determined by its size and character.

The YEAR BOOK is of considerable interest to scholars because of the reports on grants for research and to libraries for this reason and because of the section dealing with the acquisitions of the Library. In addition it contains the Charter and Laws, and lists of present and former members, and reports of committees and meetings. The YEAR BOOK is published about April 1 for the preceding calendar year. The current price is $5.00.

An author desiring to submit a manuscript for publication should send it to the Editor, George W. Corner, American Philosophical Society, 104 South Fifth Street, Philadelphia, Pa. 19106.